THE OTHER HALF OF ASPERGER SYNDROME

A guide to living in an intimate relationship with a partner who has Asperger syndrome

Maxine C. Aston

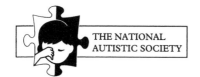

THE NATIONAL
AUTISTIC SOCIETY

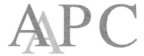

For Kevin, Zoe, Zara and William

ACKNOWLEDGEMENTS

I would like to thank all those who have helped in any way with the research and writing of this book.

In particular, I wish to thank:

- Kevin, whose part in my life gave me the determination that couples and families affected by Asperger syndrome would be offered the understanding, help and support that we sadly never received
- All the courageous partners and couples who willingly allowed me to have an insight into their lives in the hope that their knowledge and experiences could help others; without them this book could not have been written
- Brenda Wall, who has the ability to move mountains and whose constant campaigning and determination have brought about many changes and helped create an awareness of the need for a book such as this
- Dr Tony Attwood for giving me his valuable time by reading through the text and offering me his expert advice and opinions
- Dr Mark Forshaw for his comments on the original text
- Carol Darmon for giving me suggestions and proof-reading the text
- The National Autistic Society, whose staff have supported me throughout, especially Jan Snook, Chris Barson, Anne Cooper and David Potter
- Andrea Macleod of the West Midlands Autistic Society for her kind support.

Last, but definitely not least, I wish to thank my three wonderful children, Zoe, Zara and William for the strength and unselfish support that they have given me throughout my studies and the writing of this book.

PREFACE

This book has been written as a guide to Asperger syndrome for anyone who has a partner with this disorder. The information used to compile this book has been drawn from three areas – my research into this specialised area, my work as a couples counsellor and my own personal experience, having lived with a partner who was given a diagnosis of Asperger syndrome.

First published 2001 by The National Autistic Society, 393 City Road, London EC1V 1NG

ISBN 1-931282-04-8

Designed and typeset by Column Communications

CONTENTS

Contents

FOREWORD

We tend to have an image of adults with Asperger syndrome as solitary and eccentric characters, who actively avoid having an intimate relationship or desperately seek a partner, but with no success. Although this can be a description of some individuals with the syndrome, there are others who have a partner and successful career while camouflaging their disorder from their colleagues and friends. However, their partner and family can become aware of their profile of abilities, which is consistent with a diagnosis of Asperger syndrome. This book is the seminal guide to living in an intimate relationship with a partner with Asperger syndrome.

As a clinician I see many children with Asperger syndrome and I have noticed that once parents become knowledgeable regarding the characteristic profile of adults with Asperger syndrome, they scan themselves and their partner and respective families for signs of the condition. In approximately half of the families I see, it is recognised that a close adult relative to the child has a similar profile. When I subsequently see such individuals for a diagnostic assessment, one of the important discussion points is their understanding of relationships and abilities with regard to their partner.

Maxine Aston has explored the relationships of adults with Asperger syndrome as part of her academic research, as a qualified couples counsellor specialising in this area, and from her own personal relationship experience. She knows what she is writing about. She uses quotations and real examples to illustrate her points and has a compassionate understanding of both perspectives. Her insight is extraordinary and her positive attitude and strategies for successful relationships make this an essential guide for couples and counsellors.

The partners of adults with Asperger syndrome are remarkable people: they are my heroes. This book is also a tribute to their personal qualities. At last they should have the recognition they deserve and access to resources to encourage mutual understanding.

Dr Tony Attwood March 2001

The Autism Asperger Publishing Company is proud to be the sole U.S. publisher of this and a series of other carefully selected books on autism spectrum disorders originally published by the National Autistic Society (NAS) of Great Britain. To be faithful to the author, we have maintained the British spellings, punctuations, etc. We have, however, replaced a listing of sources on page 78 with U.S. equivalents in an effort to provide the most relevant and useful information to our readers.

Other NAS titles published by AAPC include:

- *Asperger Syndrome - Practical Strategies for the Classroom: A Teacher's Guide* by Leicester City Council and Leicestershire County Council
- *Challenging Behaviour and Autism: Making Sense - Making Progress: A Guide to Preventing and Managing Challenging Behaviour for Parents and Teachers* by Philip Whitaker
- *Everybody is Different: A Book for Young People Who Have Brothers or Sisters with Autism* by Fiona Bleach
- *It Can Get Better ... Dealing with Common Behaviour Problems in Young Autistic Children: A Guide to Caregivers* by Paul Dickinson and Liz Hannah
- *Teaching Young Children with Autistic Spectrum Disorders to Learn: A Practical Guide for Parents and Staff in General Education Classrooms and Preschools* by Liz Hannah
- *What is Asperger Syndrome and How Will it Affect Me? A Guide for Young People* by Martine Ives of the Autism Helpline

INTRODUCTION

This book has been written for adults who are in a close intimate relationship with someone who has either been diagnosed as having Asperger syndrome or is strongly suspected of having it.

The research for this book has taken the form of questionnaires and taped interviews that I have carried out over a period of two years. Contact with couples and partners was gained via two routes – a support group for partners of adults with Asperger syndrome and with the help and co-operation of The National Autistic Society, which mailed questionnaires to its members. A total of 35 completed questionnaires were returned. Ten of these respondents were living with or had lived with a partner who had received an official diagnosis of Asperger syndrome and, of these, five agreed to be interviewed by me. In addition, I later interviewed four adults who had received a diagnosis of Asperger syndrome. This last group consisted of three men and one woman, each of them in an intimate relationship.

I work as a trained couples counsellor and have had experience of counselling couples when one of the partners has Asperger syndrome. I have therefore had the benefit of working closely with these couples and have become aware of how unique each relationship is in terms of how it functions and operates. I have seen how many successful improvements and changes can be achieved if both partners are willing to work at their relationship and if they receive appropriate professional support and guidance.

Further, I have myself been in an intimate relationship with a man who was diagnosed as having Asperger syndrome. What I have heard and observed in other couples has therefore been deepened by my own unique and personal experience of what it is like to live in a relationship affected by this syndrome.

With two exceptions, the information in this book has been supplied by couples where the partner with Asperger syndrome is male. Therefore, there are more examples given from relationships between two such people. This is why I have also opted to use the word 'he' rather than 'she' or the long-winded 'partner who has Asperger syndrome' too frequently! Also, as a result, by 'you' I mean the woman whose male partner has the syndrome. However, those of you who are male in a relationship with a woman who has Asperger syndrome will still find the content relevant and, I hope, helpful as, fundamentally, Asperger syndrome affects males and females in the same ways. Some sections, though – particularly Initial Attraction and Parenting – contain information that is primarily applicable to women who are with a male partner who has Asperger syndrome.

There are several possible reasons for my only being able to make contact with two couples in which it is the female partner who has Asperger syndrome. Studies suggest that somewhere between 10 and 15 times more men than women are affected by Asperger syndrome.[10, 17] Another possible reason is that women generally tend to have more highly developed social and non-verbal communication skills than men, so their relationships are less likely to be problematic for their partners and the couples are less likely to ask for help. It does, however, appear that relationships are just as difficult for women with Asperger syndrome as they are for men, so the only difference may be the ways in which the partner who does not have Asperger syndrome is affected by it in the relationship.

PART I

————•◆•————

The aim of the first part of this book is to provide some basic facts about Asperger syndrome and help those without it to understand the disorder. I will also attempt to offer some insight into what brings couples together in the first place and what may lead them to the realisation that Asperger syndrome may be present in one of the partners.

Part I

SOME FACTS ABOUT ASPERGER SYNDROME

Hans Asperger and Asperger syndrome

In 1944, Hans Asperger [2] observed a pattern of behavioural problems in a group of boys while working in a Viennese clinic for disturbed children. He noted that these boys displayed an impairment in communication, both verbal and non-verbal. Their speech was inclined to be pedantic, sometimes repetitive and often quite one-sided with lengthy accounts involving the child's favourite subject. Speech was often presented in a very monotonous or overly exaggerated way, with little facial expression; jokes could be misunderstood, as could the listener's responses. The group all had deficits in eye contact and body language. Asperger described the disorder as primarily a dysfunction in social interaction. He identified this condition as 'autistic psychopathy' and believed that it was an inherited personality disorder, as he recognised similar traits in the children's parents.

Why a change of name?

Asperger syndrome has only been truly recognised in the past two decades. The name was first introduced by Lorna Wing in her classic paper published in 1981.[7] She used the name Asperger syndrome in preference to 'autistic psychopathy'. The word 'psychopathy' means an abnormality of personality and implies sociopathic behaviour – a very different disorder from what we now think of as Asperger syndrome.

What is the autistic spectrum?

Asperger syndrome is an autistic spectrum disorder. The autistic spectrum encompasses Asperger syndrome and autism, both of which may vary from severe to mild, or 'high-functioning'. Autistic spectrum disorders are also referred to as pervasive developmental disorders.

There has been much debate as to whether or not there is a difference between high-functioning autism and Asperger syndrome, both among the professionals and those with the disorders. Much literature has been written on this subject[14] and it is for each person to form their own opinions as to which name they feel is most appropriate for them.

What is Wing's triad of social and language impairments?

The criteria arrived at by Lorna Wing are now often referred to as Wing's triad of social and language impairments.[7] A diagnosis should be based on impairments in the following three areas:

- social relationships
- communication
- imagination

with a narrow, repetitive style regarding activities. There is a tendency to stick to very monotonous, fixed and seemingly dull thought patterns and behaviour.

However, to date, there is no specific universal agreement about the diagnostic criteria and Asperger syndrome did not appear in the *Diagnostic and Statistical Manual of Mental Disorders*[1], considered to be the most comprehensive and widely used reference text, until 1994.

Is Asperger syndrome hereditary?

Hans Asperger,[2] as we saw above, noticed that parents and their children had traits in common among the children he diagnosed back in the 1940s. Since then, evidence has been found for a genetic basis for Asperger syndrome, as in autism.[4] There is still much uncertainty, though, as to which particular genes, and how many, are involved.

Studies indicate that more than one gene is responsible as the severity of autism can vary drastically, even among siblings. If only one or two genes were involved, the incidence in siblings would be much higher than it is.[9] It is more likely that there is a combination of genes that determine whether or not a child is born autistic. This would explain why not all family members are affected and those who are will not always be affected to the same degree.[9]

Another complication that hinders genetic research is that, in the case of autism, as with many other medical disorders, the parents often do not have another child following the birth of an autistic child, so families are small. It is therefore impossible to know if any subsequent children would also have been autistic.[9]

Some studies have measured whether or not children diagnosed as having Asperger syndrome have a parent who has Asperger syndrome or autistic traits. One study[10] discovered that, in 57 percent of cases of children with Asperger syndrome, there was a parent who displayed autistic traits or also had Asperger syndrome. These figures do not tell us how likely it is that a couple where one partner has Asperger syndrome will have a child who will also have the syndrome. However, they do tell us that in 43 percent of cases neither parent has Asperger syndrome. This further highlights just how complex the genetic factors involved in inheritance are, and might suggest that in some cases the possibility of an environmental cause should not be ruled out.

How common is it?

A study in Sweden in 1999[12] found the prevalence figures for Asperger syndrome to be over 1 in 250. An earlier study in Sweden conducted by Ehlers and Gillberg[8] in 1993 showed the prevalence figures to be approximately 1 in 300 children. It was also discovered in the study that approximately half of the sample of the children with Asperger syndrome had not been referred for diagnosis. This study indicated that there are probably many more cases of Asperger syndrome than we are currently aware of.

IS ASPERGER SYNDROME PREDOMINANTLY A MALE CONDITION?

Statistics report more males than females

Ehlers and Gillberg[8] found that the male-to-female ratio was approximately 4:1. Clinical studies have concluded that it is much higher, suggesting ratios of between 10:1 and 15:1.[8, 10, 17] These figures, however, are only based on the people who have received a formal diagnosis – naturally, they cannot account for those among the population who have not received a diagnosis.

A partner with Asperger syndrome may be male or female

During the course of my research, I was only able to make contact with two women who have Asperger syndrome and are in an intimate long-term relationship. This is likely to be due to the fact that, as we have seen, Asperger syndrome seems to affect more males than females.[8, 10, 17] It has been estimated that one in every 250 people has Asperger syndrome and this figure alone puts the prevalence of females with Asperger syndrome at approximately one in every 1600 to 2300 individuals. Only a small proportion of adults with Asperger syndrome have an intimate sexual relationship, so it is not surprising that women with Asperger syndrome who are married or cohabiting with a sexual partner seem few and far between.

Why are females less likely to be detected?

Tony Attwood described women with Asperger syndrome as being particularly good at imitating the social actions of others and more likely to be described as immature than 'odd'.[3] This would enable a woman with Asperger syndrome to be able to learn appropriate behaviours, coping skills and strategies to deal with social situations.

The majority of the books that have been written by adults with Asperger syndrome have been written by women. This may mean that women with the syndrome are more concerned about being heard and are better able to express themselves in literature than men with it and that they wish to be acknowledged by all who care to read their valuable accounts of living with Asperger syndrome. One book in particular that highlights a woman's ability to remain undetected is by Liane Holliday Willey – *Pretending to be Normal*.[16] It offers an insider's view into being a wife and a mother with Asperger syndrome. A male reader who suspects or knows that his female partner has Asperger syndrome may gain much valuable information from reading this book.

Does gender make a difference to any problems in a relationship?

The core problems that Asperger syndrome creates for the individual are the same for women as they are for men, so most of the information given in this book will apply to both sexes. The extent to which a particular individual is affected and how they deal with the problems that having Asperger syndrome can cause, however, will vary between males and females. This can be explained by the fact that Asperger syndrome seems to exaggerate some of the difficulties that some men may already have with verbal and non-verbal communication.

It has been claimed that women are superior to men at interpreting positive non-verbal information,[13] which may give women an automatic advantage in the area of social skills and communication. It is therefore possible for a woman with Asperger syndrome to have a greater ability to conceal the emotional and social problems she may be experiencing in her everyday life than would a man with the syndrome. The advantages that women have regarding social skills could make it harder to detect Asperger syndrome in the more able woman, and if she has learned good social strategies and coping skills, her partner may remain unaware of its presence. He may even find the lack of emotion an advantage in their relationship, especially if they share the same special interest.

Why the apparent increase in the numbers of men with Asperger syndrome?

It is also more likely that you are married to or living with a male, rather than a female, partner with Asperger syndrome. It does appear that the syndrome is predominantly a male condition.[2, 8]

So why does it seem that, all of a sudden, more men are being diagnosed as having Asperger syndrome? Besides the obvious reason that awareness of

Asperger syndrome has increased greatly over the past two decades, making it more likely that if you have the syndrome this will be recognised, it is also possible that, in the past, the behaviour of men with Asperger syndrome was more likely to be overlooked than it is today. The more able men with the syndrome who do seek out relationships are often very hard and conscientious workers, so they are often also good providers. In view of these dispositions, their problems with social interaction may have been conveniently overlooked in the past, as the financial support offered by these men was possibly considered more important to their wives then than how they related to them on an emotional level.

Today, however, women are asking for better emotional interaction and a deeper level of communication with their partners. They are no longer prepared to accept the 'women feel and men think' view. Most women expect understanding, intimacy and emotional support from their partner; they want to be able to express their feelings and be understood.

Equally, the financial status of women in our society is changing rapidly, with employers recognising women's potential in terms of careers and increasing flexibility in the job market. With the rise in the numbers of jobs available to women and the increase in women's capacity to earn, the traditional dependence on a man as the sole financial supporter has, for some women, decreased. As women become more independent, they ask for support in more areas than just the financial side of the relationship. Most women want more from their partners than just money; they want to feel loved and appreciated.

All these factors may explain why more men with Asperger syndrome are being identified today. Women are not keeping quiet and they are recognising that their partners are not simply being 'just like a man'. Thus, the numbers of men with Asperger syndrome may simply have increased because their problems with social interaction are no longer being sidelined.

SUSPECTED, UNDIAGNOSED ASPERGER SYNDROME

The first step

I received almost three times as many replies from respondents who strongly suspected their partner had Asperger syndrome than I did from those with a partner who had been diagnosed. The journey of discovery for those who are uncertain as to whether or not their partners have it can be confusing and sometimes ambiguous. One of the aims of this book is to offer some guidance and attempt to clarify some

17

of the doubts that you may have if you are in this situation.

There are various reasons that might lead you to wonder if your partner has Asperger syndrome. It may be that you have seen an article in a magazine or newspaper or it could be that there has been a programme on the radio or television about it. Asperger syndrome is being mentioned more and more in the media and so knowing about it may lead to you thinking that your partner could have the syndrome. Alternatively, you might have a child who has been diagnosed as having Asperger syndrome or autism. Such awareness of autistic spectrum disorders may provoke the realisation that there are similarities between your child's behaviour and your partner's. Equally, if you are an adult with undiagnosed Asperger syndrome, you may even recognise for yourself that you have problems in the same areas as your child.

The paradoxical nature of Asperger syndrome

A person living with a partner who has Asperger syndrome may have been aware for many years that something is not quite right, and perhaps have a sense of something being missing or not fitting into place. Someone who is in a sexual relationship with another is more likely than anyone else to know him on a very intimate and personal level. She will be very aware of what a paradox her partner is: so capable in some areas, yet so disabled in others and unable to understand what it is he does, or fails to do, that can cause both himself and his partner so many problems and misunderstandings.

Asperger syndrome can make a more capable high achiever seem just such a paradox. It can give many mixed and ambiguous messages that can lead to a lot of confused emotions for the person living with him.

A person with Asperger syndrome may be an expert in a particular, often obscure, field – Edwardian architecture, computers, aircraft, automobiles, theology, music or something bizarre such as the shapes of electric pylons or empty cleaning cartons. He will know his chosen field of interest inside out. His rote memory can be amazing and his ability to recall facts and figures will defy all logic, especially as they often seem to acquire all this knowledge without any effort. He may be able to do all these things and often be very competent at them and yet many women have said they have not felt able to leave their partner in charge of the children, for fear that there would be some unpredicted crisis and their partner would have difficulty coping with it.

OBSESSIVE BEHAVIOUR OR SPECIAL INTERESTS?

Routines can be rigid and precise

A person with Asperger syndrome may have many rigid daily routines, and it may have been these that first made his partner notice that this was not usual behaviour, not something you would expect a person to engage in. It could be that mealtimes have to be very precise, always served at the same time every day, and certain foods have to be cooked in a certain way. Many different routines have been identified in adults with Asperger syndrome, and how closely these have to be observed will vary from person to person. When a routine has become firmly established, everyone will have to fit in with it; any form of change is likely to cause mayhem. This fixed regime can make something quite simple, like going out for a meal, into hard work and certainly not the enjoyable experience it should be.

These strict routines can include door and window locking, turning off the gas, mealtimes, only eating certain foods, only using certain cleaning materials, taking certain routes in the car and many more. You might have thought initially that your partner was just being awkward, but there is a chance that, before this particular disorder was suspected, the behaviour may have been attributed to a condition called obsessive compulsive disorder (OCD).

Asperger syndrome and obsessive compulsive disorder

OCD can often manifest itself in the form of repetitive behaviours similar to those already described. Obsessions with cleaning and checking have been identified in cases of Asperger syndrome and these can be easily confused with OCD when there is not a full awareness of the diagnostic criteria for Asperger syndrome. In some cases, OCD can occur independently in someone who has Asperger syndrome and this would be for a clinical psychologist or psychiatrist to assess. They are certainly not the same thing.

More to Asperger syndrome than just obsessions

Asperger syndrome does not end there – it is not just about having obsessions or routines. To receive a diagnosis of Asperger syndrome requires that other areas of life are also affected. Those with the syndrome will have problems with communication and it may be difficult for them to engage in a very deep, meaningful conversation about their partners' feelings and how those feelings affect the relationship. There will be problems in reading non-verbal signals, such as facial expressions and body language, and also in being able to give the right responses when talking. Many women have said that they did not feel necessary to their partners on an emotional level and that they were needed more for what they did than for who they were and how they felt.

Not just a case of men being men

Especially when the partner with Asperger syndrome is male, some may argue that this is just the way some men are and that women have always been better mindreaders than men. Asperger syndrome, though, is something very different, and partners may sense that this is not just a case of their men just being 'typical men'.

You may also sense that there is a deeper problem than your partner just being awkward because something about his responses and actions shows that he is uncertain about what to do or how you are expecting him to respond. This may lead you to think at times that it is you who are unable to make yourself understood and that the problem in communicating lies with you.

Questioning your sanity

Many women have reported that they felt they were going completely mad. They could not understand why their partners were unable to comprehend what they were trying to tell them, and why they would accuse them of criticising every time they tried to help or offer some advice. Some women felt they were becoming 'nags' because they ended up repeating the same things over and over again and found themselves in the same locked situation with their partners.

Can things change? The answer is 'yes'. However, without knowledge of the disorder, it may be you who is doing most of the changing. Initially, some women reported that they tried to suppress what they felt in order to deal with what their partners were doing in a less emotional way. They tried to avoid certain situations and topics, especially those involving some sort of social interaction.

SOCIALISING, FRIENDS, PRESENT AND PAST

Social situations

There is the strong possibility that social situations involving the couple will have, in some instances, become embarrassing or highly stressful for you. One woman described visiting the local supermarket with her partner for their weekly shopping. She reported the feelings of utter embarrassment she experienced when her partner insisted on lining up all the cans on the conveyor belt in a precise symmetrical way, completely oblivious to the long queue of impatient shoppers forming behind them.

Another couple held a party and her partner went to bed. Even worse was the experience of a woman who described the feeling of horror she felt when a friend asked her what she thought of her new outfit. Her partner, who was standing with her, answered instead and gave her his honest opinion. He also recommended that if she lost a few pounds it might be an improvement!

Friends

The behaviour of a person with Asperger syndrome may at times appear rude, especially to those who are not aware of the disorder. So, it may not come as too much of a surprise to find that a person with the syndrome does not always have any real friends. What may be surprising, however, is that they seem to have never had any friends, and do not appear to have really needed any.

There may be different reasons for the fact that there has been a lack of friends. One may be that they simply never wanted any and were always too absorbed in some hobby or simply chose very solitary pursuits. In the case of more able partners with Asperger syndrome, it is more likely that they have always wanted friends – probably quite desperately at times – and may have wondered why, whenever they tried to make friends, they never seemed to get it quite right. Women with Asperger syndrome may have tried taking on different personas to try and fit in with peer groups. The problems with forming friendships will go right back to childhood.

Asperger syndrome is lifelong

Asperger syndrome is present from birth – it is not something that develops in later life and it will not go away. It is not the result of childhood or adult trauma, nor is it the result of abuse or emotional neglect or rejection by cold parents who could not express their emotions.

It is not always detected in the early years and may even go unrecognised until adolescence or adulthood. Adolescence is often a very bewildering and intensely traumatic time for those with Asperger syndrome. It can leave them feeling that they were treated quite unfairly as a child and teenager, especially if, like many children with Asperger syndrome, they were bullied at school.

The effect of childhood bullying and Asperger syndrome

Bullying can have an adverse affect on all children. It can lower their self-esteem, confidence and ability to be assertive. To children with Asperger syndrome, bullying can often go unreported and undetected and the lessons it teaches about other people can live with them all their lives. They can carry with them the belief that others are out to trick them, make fun of them and make them look stupid. This can exaggerate their reaction to perceived criticisms of themselves and it is this heightened sensitivity that their partner may experience first hand when trying to discuss how they feel about a particular issue.

TRYING TO COMMUNICATE

Taking things literally

Problems with literal and double meanings can cause many misunderstandings for those with Asperger syndrome, many of whom complain that they wish people would just say what they mean.

In a couple where one partner has not yet been diagnosed as having Asperger syndrome, the other partner can feel quite bewildered and at times infuriated that he cannot understand what she is trying to say and often seems to completely miss the point. Some women say that they do not see why something so simple should cause such chaos. One woman explained how she had told her husband she would 'kill him' if he forgot to pick up the dry cleaning in his lunch hour. She was going to speak at an important conference and needed the outfit that was at the cleaners for that evening. He forgot to collect it and took her threat to kill him quite seriously, so he was too afraid to go home. She eventually received a call from her sister-in-law to say that he had phoned her because he was concerned that if he returned home he was in danger of losing his life.

As well as misunderstandings over the literal meanings in communication, non-verbal communication between the two halves of the couple may also cause problems.

Giving non-verbal messages

It can be difficult for those with Asperger syndrome to get facial expressions right, and knowing when to smile can be one of the problems. You may be telling your partner something quite serious and important, but when you glance at him, he smiles, leaving you thinking, 'What is he smiling about?'

Eye movements may also appear odd, your partner perhaps staring for too long or looking away at an inappropriate moment. This lack of co-ordination with others' facial expressions can also show itself in body language.

Body language and personal space

Some with Asperger syndrome do not have the natural ability to learn the unwritten rules regarding personal space that others take for granted. They will sometimes stand where they want to stand and seem unaware that they may be standing too close to someone. This can give strange and sometimes threatening signals to someone who is not aware of the reasons behind this behaviour.

Hand movements can sometimes be non-existent or exaggerated. People with Asperger syndrome may walk in a slightly odd way: their movements may be quite stiff, their arms swinging in a kind of regimented way or perhaps there might be a clumsiness to their movements. There may also be an awkwardness or oddness to the way in which they take part in conversations. Their facial expression has been described by some women as 'wooden'. Eye contact can be evasive and this can sometimes give the impression that there is a lack of honesty or openness, which is not the case at all. When you know that the person has Asperger syndrome, these problematic issues in communication can be explained and understood.

SEEKING A DIAGNOSIS

Making the decision to be assessed

A couple need to give very careful consideration to the question of whether or not they should seek out a diagnosis.

If one partner does not want to accept or investigate the possibility of Asperger syndrome, the other partner has to decide how important it is to them and if they can live without having a formal diagnosis. Whatever they decide, it must be the decision of the person who may have Asperger syndrome to go and seek a referral, and the other partner should not try to force the situation either way. He/she should reach this decision in his own time, when he/she is ready to face it, and feels prepared and willing to accept a possible positive diagnosis. After all, it is no small thing to face the possibility of finding out that he/she has a lifelong disorder that cannot be cured.

On the positive side, receiving a diagnosis can offer the opportunity for the person to learn specific skills and make improvements in his/her personal and professional life.

The importance of being aware

Having a diagnosis can make a great deal of difference to the couple's relationship as it brings an awareness of the effects of Asperger syndrome on the couple. Awareness, followed by acceptance, is the first step towards dealing with them effectively.

Even if the adult who may have Asperger syndrome does not wish to go for an assessment, as long as they are aware that it may be the cause of some of their problems, the couple will be able to move forward and work on the difficulties they are facing. If, however, the partner who may have Asperger syndrome is unwilling to accept that he may have a disorder and blames everything or everyone else for the problems in the relationship, then it will be very difficult for the relationship to survive. Sometimes the blame can be directed at the partner without Asperger syndrome and this can have a devastating effect on both them and the relationship.

Seeking a referral

If you as a couple decide to seek a referral, this can be done by both of you visiting your GP and discussing it or if you can afford it, you may prefer to seek private advice. If at all possible it is important to check that the psychiatrist or clinical psychologist to whom you are referred is informed about or specialises in Asperger syndrome. Although professionals are becoming more knowledgeable in this area, there are still many who do not yet fully understand what having Asperger syndrome implies and how to recognise and diagnose it correctly.

Medical health workers sometimes link Asperger syndrome with severe autism and have very misguided and preconceived ideas about what being on the autistic spectrum entails. One myth, for instance, is that adults with Asperger syndrome do not form sexual relationships or marry, which is clearly not the case.

It is helpful for you as a couple to go together to see your GP as the partner without Asperger syndrome may be able to provide valuable information and give the other partner support. Just a short consultation with a GP will not be enough to enable him or her to make a decision as to whether or not one partner has Asperger syndrome, so a referral to a clinical psychologist or psychiatrist should be offered.

Coming to a diagnosis

Different psychiatrists and clinical psychologists may use various methods to arrive at a diagnosis. It is very helpful if both partners go to the appointment together as the more information that can be provided the better, especially any details about the developmental history of the person with suspected Asperger syndrome. These last details are very important to help form an accurate diagnosis, and questions will be asked about childhood, parents and siblings, any problems at school or work, adolescence, friendships and relationships. Information about hobbies, special interests and routines will also be asked for, as well as life within the family and any other particular areas that may be problematic.

A positive diagnosis

If a couple has reached the stage of a consultation, it is very possible that there will be a positive diagnosis of Asperger syndrome. However prepared you both are for being told that one of you has Asperger syndrome, it will almost always have an impact. You may feel relieved initially or completely numb.

The partner with Asperger syndrome, on the other hand, could appear completely unaffected. One woman described how her partner was more impressed by the fact the psychiatrist had the same tie on as he did than he was by being told that he had Asperger syndrome. It is therefore important not to presume that your partner will feel unduly disturbed or horrified by the diagnosis. It is also a good idea for each of you to say how you feel about the diagnosis and not to make any assumptions for each other.

AFTER THE DIAGNOSIS, WHAT NEXT?

Acceptance

After receiving a diagnosis of Asperger syndrome, you need to give yourselves time to accept it. Although for some it may seem unfair or a hopeless situation when they discover for certain that their partner has Asperger syndrome, it can also come as quite a revelation. It can help to make sense of many of the things that were hard to understand about a partner's behaviour and explain some of the problems that have hindered the relationship.

Once you know that Asperger syndrome has been responsible for some of the problems you have been having, you can extend your knowledge and understanding of the disorder. You can work out better strategies for dealing with these problematic areas. There is no cure for Asperger syndrome – no magic pill or remedy to put it right – and a lot of hard work and changes will be required by both partners, but especially by the partner without Asperger syndrome.

You will both have to decide who you are going to tell and how to explain what Asperger syndrome is. Some people may find it difficult to understand or accept. Others may, wrongfully, view it as a mental illness and be fearful, thinking that it makes your partner odd or different, someone to be wary of. It is important that whoever is told receives an adequate explanation of what Asperger syndrome is. Tell them that it is a developmental disorder that causes problems in specific areas (social interaction and communication, obsessive tendencies and a need for routine) and that, in other respects, your partner is capable and no different from anyone else. The main thing is that your partner should be treated with the same amount of respect and dignity as any other human being.

The end of the journey to discovery

After receiving a diagnosis, as the partner without Asperger syndrome, you may be left feeling both happy and sad. Although you are likely to feel a sense of relief and that you now have the ability to understand what has been causing many of the problems in the relationship, you may also feel like you have reached the end of a journey and be rather exhausted by it all.

You will very likely be in need of some comforting. The trouble is that your partner may not be aware of this need or be able to offer this kind of support and warmth. Tell your partner how you feel but not in a judgmental way: this is not about blame. Explain in a direct and clear way that you are relieved you now both know the reason why there have been some problems in the relationship and that together you can now work at sorting things out. If possible, do this when you are both sitting quietly together, have plenty of time and will not be interrupted.

One woman I spoke to had an agreement with her husband that, rather than expecting him automatically to know, she would always tell him when she wanted a hug. This took the pressure away from him and he was always happy to oblige. If your partner, though, is not able to offer any comfort, then it is important to seek support from friends and family who can prove quite invaluable at this time.

Feelings of loss

There may be a sense of loss at this time, almost a feeling that something has died. This is not surprising – something *has* died. The relationship as it was perceived before the diagnosis is no more and you now know that things will never be quite the same again.

You know that all the tactics and ways that have been used to try and change things in the past have been ineffective and you will have to start all over again with new ones.

You may feel that you no longer know the person you fell in love with.

For all these and other reasons, it is often the partner without Asperger syndrome who is left with a sense of loss. This time can feel quite lonely as it is unlikely that your partner will be able to empathise with you or share these feelings.

Feelings of anger

Sometimes there can be a feeling of anger once a diagnosis of Asperger syndrome has been accepted for your partner. You may feel you have been cheated out of having a normal relationship or that you have spent years trying to achieve something that was never going to be possible.

The feelings of anger may not be directed at anybody in particular but they may be aimed at your partner's parents, life, God, the professionals or something else. There can be a need for a scapegoat and so your anger may be directed at your partner, despite the fact that it is not his fault he has Asperger syndrome. This can be disruptive and negative for both of you.

In time, the anger will burn out. Only then should you start to make decisions about what to do and where to go from there. Rash decisions made while you are still in the middle of this angry phase will be short-lived and probably quite negative, so it is important to take things easy until the anger subsides.

Where to go from here

Some women report feeling like getting out altogether and starting a new life. If you do decide to do this, then it is important that you do not feel like a deserter who has abandoned a sinking ship. It is not everybody who can live with the absence of intimate communication, reciprocated feelings and empathy that, to a greater or lesser extent, are part of Asperger syndrome.

Before the diagnosis, which brings with it the realisation that Asperger syndrome is the cause of some of the problems, you may have kept struggling to bring about changes in the relationship and lived in the hope that things could and would change. Hope can keep people going through many adverse situations. With a diagnosis or acceptance that a partner has Asperger syndrome, however, that hope might feel as if it has been wiped out. This does not have to be the case – your goals just have to become realistic. Indeed, many relationships where one partner has Asperger syndrome are successful.

Hope can live on

If you are the partner without Asperger syndrome, a diagnosis gives you two positive pieces of information:

- you now know that you are not going crazy
- your partner did not mean to upset you by some of things he did or did not do.

Women report many instances that they had found hurtful before receiving a positive diagnosis, such as a birthday card signed like a business letter, not being visited in hospital by their partner because hospitals make them feel uneasy, being abandoned at a party or feeling let down by their partner's reluctance to share in an intimate moment. Often they have found that, afterwards, they are able to understand some of these things that had previously left them feeling upset or bewildered. Things that had happened that they could not understand before started to make sense and fall into place.

Some women, though, were left wondering why they did not realise earlier what was causing the problems and why they turned a blind eye to the obvious fact that this was not just selfish or awkward behaviour by their partner, that there was something more at work. The next chapter sets out to explain why some of these signs are unconsciously ignored and what it is that attracted you to your partner in the first place.

INITIAL ATTRACTION

Kind, gentle men

This section is written for women who have a male partner with Asperger syndrome, as I do not have sufficient data regarding what attracts men to women who have the syndrome. However, it appears likely from the information I do have, that a woman with Asperger syndrome will seek out someone who is likely to be a reliable and steady father figure, does not make strong emotional or intimate demands on her and allows her a lot of freedom and autonomy in the relationship.

Most of the women with male partners with the syndrome describe them as being very kind, gentle and quiet men when they first met them and these were the characteristics that they were initially attracted to. These men can display a naiveté that has a boyish essence to it, and the women they often choose have strong maternal, caring and warm ways. So, almost instantly, there can be a 'fit' between the two halves of a couple of this type.

The feminine side of Asperger syndrome

Boys with Asperger syndrome are sometimes taunted at school because they adopt a somewhat feminine approach and are less likely to conform to social stereotypes of masculine and feminine behaviour than is the case with their peers. Their mother is more likely to be their role model than their father, because it is often the mother they spend more time with. This could lead to boys displaying mannerisms and gestures that could be misinterpreted by other children as being 'gay'; name-calling and bullying could be the consequence.

Such a feminine side in an adult male can be very appealing to some women. Many men with Asperger syndrome are quite happy to cook, clean, iron and even flower arrange if they so wish. They do not feel obligated to fulfil and display masculine roles, but are much more likely to do what pleases them, rather than what society states they are supposed to do. They can have quite a gentle approach and rarely display aggressive behaviour. Many women interpret this as meaning that they are sure enough of their masculinity to be in touch with their feminine side as well. They see this as a positive quality in a partner.

As men with Asperger syndrome often choose women who are quite strong, independent and nurturing, this all fits together very well for a while. It is only after a time together that the contradiction of this feminine side emerges. Although he can be gentle, he can also begin to display some rather chauvinistic traits. His chosen partner may be expected to fill a certain role and that role may depend on his mother. He may expect things done for him exactly as she did for him. It is possible that he chose his partner because she was in some way like his mother, and there is a possibility that she may be older than he is.

An older woman

It is not the case that men with Asperger syndrome deliberately search out older women. However, many of the women I encountered in the course of my research were older than their male partners. This finding differs from most of the existing literature on couples, which indicates that it is far more likely that the male will be older than the female.

One of the theories proposed to explain this is that a man will exchange his wealth for a woman's youth and attractiveness. This rule does not seem to apply when the man in a relationship has Asperger syndrome and this can feel very flattering for a woman living in a society where youth and looks seem to govern so many men's choices of female partners. It may be that age is not too important to someone who has Asperger syndrome, as they often appear not to discriminate on the basis of a person's age or status. It may also be that men with Asperger syndrome prefer, and feel more comfortable with, an older woman and have decided that age equates to maternal and nurturing ways.

Hard workers and good providers

Another reason for attraction may be that the more able men with Asperger syndrome are often highly qualified and have very well-paid jobs – frequently within the fields of engineering, science, mathematics or computing. The ability to work with objects rather than people could be described as a characteristic trait of Asperger syndrome.

Simon Baron-Cohen[5] described individuals with Asperger syndrome as being highly capable in the area of 'folk physics', which is understanding objects, and quite poor in the area of 'folk psychology', which is understanding people and their thoughts. Thus, unfortunately, when they have to deal with other people – whether it is management, other employees or the public – they can face major problems, unless they are fortunate enough to work in very liberal surroundings or solitary conditions. However, some employers will often overlook the social problems an adult with the syndrome displays as their hard and conscientious work compensates for it.

Interests in common?

There may be similar interests or a particular hobby shared by the couple. Love of the theatre, politics, religion and, in particular, music have all been mentioned as shared common interests that brought a couple together.

Sometimes, though, the special interest is not always as straightforward as it might first appear. One woman reported that she had been attracted to her husband because of his Christian beliefs. He said he was interested in the Bible, but you can imagine her surprise when he proudly showed her his collection of hundreds of bibles. Another woman was pleased to have found someone who shared her interest in classical music. In fact, her new partner seemed quite an expert on the composers – so much so that she eventually realised this was his one and only topic of conversation. As long as they discussed music and composers, things were fine, but beyond that it was as though he had absolutely nothing to say to her. Music was his obsession.

Obsessive love

Women have reported that they eventually realised that *they* were their partner's obsession a little while after they started seeing each other. It would be difficult for most people not to feel flattered by so much attention and devotion from someone just wanting to please them and spend all their time with them. It is no wonder that many women feel important, special and needed at this time.

Most people want to feel needed, but there is a difference between being needed and totally depended on, which is what this need can gradually become. It is this obsessive love, appealing and attractive in the beginning, that eventually becomes the very thing that can drive the two people in the relationship apart.

You may feel like the responsibility for the whole relationship is weighing on your shoulders.

Whirlwind romance

Some women talked about having gone through quite a short, whirlwind romance that moved rapidly through the stages of courtship and on to marriage. Courtship with men with Asperger syndrome can be short-lived if their sole desire is to find a wife. Often it is a need to be married that motivates men with Asperger syndrome to seek out a partner in the first place. If such a man believes he has found a suitable partner who has all the qualities he is looking for, then the topic of marriage may enter the conversation quite early on.

Love is blind

'Love is blind', they say, and this is especially true of the early stages of a relationship. It is not uncommon to focus on and exaggerate a new-found partner's positive qualities. Women can think, 'Here is this caring and (possibly) handsome man, with a good, respectable, well-paid job, who is honest, kind and gentle – I'm so lucky.' They ignore the fact that their friends or family find him a little bit eccentric or different, or that misunderstandings and communication problems are occurring.

Some women turn a blind eye when, for instance, their partner insists on being in charge of planning all their outings or journeys, sometimes in great detail. One woman described how her husband even insisted on teaching her the 'correct way' of putting the rubbish in the bin. In the early days of the relationship, many women decide they can live with these unusual little ways, but it can become increasingly difficult to do so as time goes on.

After the honeymoon

Some women have talked about feeling that, once they entered into marriage, their partner stopped trying – the romance ended and so did the feeling of being important and special to him. Some felt that, all of a sudden, their husband's efforts to please them stopped and he simply returned to his former lifestyle. Suddenly these women found themselves being expected to fit in with all their partner's needs for routine and a schedule, tolerate his special interests and not have a social life, intimate communication and, in some cases, sex.

Fulfilling a need

Some women described this time as particularly difficult as they tried to understand their partner's needs. They did not want to give up and walk out and, when talking failed, many tried to change themselves and began to question their own sanity. Some women described it as feeling like they were not being appreciated for who they were and, no matter how hard they tried, communication constantly broke down. They could feel themselves getting more and more angry and frustrated as they tried to make sense of things and understand just what it was that somehow kept leading them back to the same place. Some talked about having a feeling that something was missing, like the last piece needed to complete a jigsaw, and the sense that they were there simply to fulfil their partner's needs rather than there being the necessary give and take.

Being stuck in this very painful situation and feeling bewildered and confused can sometimes go on for months or, in many cases, years before the couple discovers what is wrong. Some women reported going to their doctors and being recommended for couples counselling or sometimes the couples arranged to go for counselling themselves. This is an avenue many couples find themselves travelling down when one of the partners has Asperger syndrome.

GETTING HELP

Couples counselling

Receiving couples counselling when relationships have run into problems can, in many cases, help to revive them. Indeed, the problems in many marriages and relationships have been solved within a counselling room. Unfortunately, this does not often appear to be the case when one partner has Asperger syndrome.

For some, the result has been disastrous, leaving the partner who does not have Asperger syndrome feeling unheard, frustrated and very angry. The reason for this is likely to be that the presence of Asperger syndrome has not been recognised by either the couple or the counsellor. However, from my own work as a couples counsellor, I know that this need not be the case.

When there is an awareness that one of you has Asperger syndrome and the counsellor is experienced in this area, counselling can be a very positive and rewarding experience for both partners. Couples have been able to achieve many successful changes by using suitable coping skills and strategies. Counselling can help sift through the problem areas and identify what is due to the partner having Asperger syndrome and what is not. The result is that the couple can feel better equipped to deal with problems and each can feel more appreciated and understood by the other. You will feel listened to, validated and supported in your attempts to maintain and strengthen the relationship, which means a lot.

When a couple seeks counselling, it is quite possible that neither partner knows that one of them has Asperger syndrome. This alone can mean that counselling will not work. If, at a later date, one of them receives a positive diagnosis, the counsellor may be held responsible by the couple for not knowing at the time that this was the problem and acting on it. However, counsellors are not psychologists, nor are they psychiatrists, so they are unlikely to have been trained to recognise a complex condition such as Asperger syndrome. Nor are counsellors qualified to make an official diagnosis, and the ethics surrounding this are very precise.

If counsellors do suspect that clients have Asperger syndrome, they can suggest that they contact The National Autistic Society and seek further information for themselves. Alternatively, they could both visit their GP to seek a referral to a psychiatrist for a clinical assessment.

Once the couple has sought professional medical advice and investigated the possibility of the presence of Asperger syndrome, they can return to counselling once again.

Seeking specialist help

When a couple knows that one of the them has Asperger syndrome, they should request that they receive appropriate specialised counselling for the problems that they are facing. This is one of the gains of having sought and received a diagnosis. Both partners will feel understood and that their concerns are being heard if they see a counsellor who specialises in this area and is familiar with the effects the syndrome can have on the couple's relationship.

The importance of having counsellors specially trained to help people in this situation is slowly being recognised. At the moment, there are few counsellors who are able to offer specialist counselling to couples in this situation (again, see the section at the back of the book). Hopefully, as awareness of the need for this kind of support grows, its availability will improve in the near future.

Part I

PART II

———•———

The aim in the second part of this book is to look at some of the problems that living with a partner who has Asperger syndrome can present. In the pages that follow are various strategies and ways of coping with difficulties that have worked for others. Most of these apply equally to women who have a male partner with Asperger syndrome and men who have a female partner with the syndrome. It is, though, impossible to generalise and what works for one couple will not necessarily work for another as each individual and relationship is unique, so see what works best for you.

LIVING AND COPING WITH ASPERGER SYNDROME

Each of us is unique

Every human being is unique, just as every couple's relationship is unique. That said, when one partner has Asperger syndrome, all couples for whom this is the case will have something in common with each other.

Having the syndrome will result in a similar set of problems being created within any relationship with a member of the opposite sex. How severe these problems are and how they affect each couple will be dependent on an accumulation of factors. One of these will be how well you are able to cope and find better ways in which to deal with problems as they arise. Another important factor will be how severely your partner is affected by the syndrome and in what particular areas he is disabled.

The fact that your partner has formed a long-term intimate relationship with you is a very positive thing as it is likely to mean that he is at the higher, more able end of the spectrum. Many adults with Asperger syndrome never form such relationships. For some this is because they are not interested in developing them, while for others the desire is there, but they have neither the social skills nor ability to do so. Finally, for some adults with Asperger syndrome, there can be little motivation to change. They can therefore remain quite rigid within their particular lifestyles or ways, so their relationships do not develop and are prone to fading out very quickly.

Not everyone with Asperger syndrome is the same

Once again, because every person is unique, having Asperger syndrome will affect each person in a very individual way. There will be problems with communication, socialising and imaginative thought, but how this manifests will vary from person to person.

It may be that their lives are not full of obsessive interests or rigid routines because not all higher-functioning adults with Asperger syndrome have obvious obsessive tendencies. You may not find that there are major problems over socialising in your relationship, but trying to get your views across could prove impossible.

Your partner may not want to talk about feelings and emotions, but that does not mean he does not have any. Many varied factors will play their part in how each person is affected, such as their age, upbringing, capacity for learning and, most importantly, the person they have chosen to share their life with.

A social guide

If you are in an intimate relationship with someone who has Asperger syndrome, you are one of the most important people in their lives. How you approach and cope with problems can make a difference to how he copes with many of the difficulties that having Asperger syndrome can present him with. This is not to say that you will have to take responsibility for everything your partner does, but it is important that you are aware that there are some things that you will be naturally better at than he is.

You will have a strong advantage over your partner in the area of social skills, interaction and communication, and this may be even more the case if your partner is male. In many ways, a person with Asperger syndrome is socially myopic and will rely on you to be their guide in a society that must at times be very confusing.

It is wise to know what problems are likely to occur as a direct result of your partner having Asperger syndrome and what it is he actually can make choices about. One area that my research has pinpointed as being particularly problematic in a relationship is that of communication between partners and other family members, so this is the subject of the next section.

IMPROVING COMMUNICATION

Difficulties with communication

Communication seems to be the one area that many women cite as being the most problematic in their relationship. This is not surprising considering that difficulties with both verbal and non-verbal forms of communication are strongly indicative, together with other criteria, of Asperger syndrome.

Communication problems arising when living with a partner who has Asperger syndrome can drive some adults into a state of despair and desperation. Women have described this as feeling like they and their partner 'come from different cultures' or are 'talking in different languages.' Trying to find some way of getting a particular point across to your partner can lead to frustration, anger and utter despair.

Reasons for these misunderstandings can vary from couple to couple. Maybe your partner has a problem with distinguishing the literal from sarcasm, a joke, figure of speech or whatever and so will interpret most of what is being said in the literal sense of the words. Maybe he finds instructions hard to understand and you find yourself repeating the same things over and over again. It could be that he simply does not get the point of what is being said. Something that may appear quite obvious to you will not necessarily be obvious to your partner, and some very awkward and infuriating misunderstandings can develop between you because of this.

Maybe your partner reacts very quickly with anger to something that appears quite trivial, leaving you feeling rejected and dismissed. Perhaps he appears to have a very selective memory, only seeming to remember a part of what has been said and then taking it completely out of context. Maybe he just interprets everything that has been said as criticism when, most of the time, all that is being offered is some practical advice.

Whatever form these crossed wires take, it is almost guaranteed that there will be problems with verbal and non-verbal communication between partners in a couple when one of you has Asperger syndrome.

Good communication is vital

Good-quality communication between both partners in a couple is very important. Too many misunderstandings in the relationship can cause it to begin to break down and show signs of stress. As well as misunderstandings, if there is an almost total absence of communication, this can be very destructive. Not being heard or acknowledged can be as distressing as being verbally abused.

How something is said and the body language that accompanies it are just as important as what is being said if each of you is to understand what the other is saying. Eye contact, body language and facial expression can help smooth out two-way interactions, and if they do not run smoothly, confusion is inevitable.

Many people with Asperger syndrome show impairment in non-verbal communication skills and often have difficulties with the 'pragmatics of speech'. Non-verbal communication refers to the non-verbal signals we give while talking, such as facial expressions and body language, that expand on and clarify what we are saying in words. The way we position our body, our posture and gestures can be valuable indicators as to how we feel and the message we convey to another person. We also put emphasis on particular words and change our tone of voice to convey the meaning of what is being said – these cues are called the pragmatics of speech.

A person with Asperger syndrome will have difficulty with both reading non-verbal and pragmatic signs and sending them. For instance, someone who can look a person in the eye and talk with confidence is likely to be perceived as honest. If your partner does not get these important signals right, you may think he is being evasive or untruthful.

Ambiguity and Asperger syndrome do not mix

If these two ingredients are put together, then it can result in an instant disaster. It is very important to be precise, direct and straight to the point if your partner has Asperger syndrome. This is because he will not always understand double meanings, nor automatically know what had *not* been meant. One woman told her husband that if he did not change he would have to leave and, much to her horror, the next day he left. He took it that that was what she really meant and wanted and, as he did not feel he could change, he left. He could not see that, at the time, she was upset and was desperately trying to get a response out of him that would prompt him to change some of his ways and that she did not really want him to go.

Ordinarily, this would not happen as a partner would know that most people say things when they are upset or angry that they do not necessarily mean. Unfortunately, someone with Asperger syndrome may find underlying meanings very difficult to understand, so it is important that you remember to say what you mean and mean what you say – this alone can prevent many misunderstandings. Sometimes, though, it can make conversing very tiring and lengthy, especially when you are feeling fed up and just wish that your partner would understand the point of what is being said. At such times, it would be best to take a break and come back to the topic later on. Whatever course you take, it is certainly worthwhile remaining clear and precise, as this will make life far easier in the long run.

It is not a case of being awkward

Before knowing about Asperger syndrome, many people may suspect their partners of just being awkward or not trying or wanting to interact and communicate effectively. Once a positive diagnosis has been received, you then know that your partner is not being deliberately evasive or uncommunicative. It is not because he does not *want* to understand what is being said, it is much more likely that he simply does not understand it.

As we have seen, having the syndrome can mean that communication is very difficult if what is being said is not framed in a clear and precise way. This does not mean that your partner is not intelligent and does not have the ability to learn – indeed, it is likely that he will have a higher than average IQ.

If he is given the correct help, support and guidance and has the motivation to learn, he can develop strategies to help him cope and respond appropriately in communication and social situations.

Your partner is not stupid!

The only type of intelligence affected by Asperger syndrome is social intelligence.

It is likely that your partner has been made to feel stupid many times in his life. As a child, he is likely to have been singled out, identified as 'different' and bullied at school. The bullying was probably quite severe and so, as an adult, he may be very sensitive to any form of perceived ridicule or put-down, especially from you. This could instantly anger him and he may react to the situation as if he were suddenly back in the playground, placing you on the outside, as a foe.

Once this happens, there is very little chance that you will be able to reach a reconciliation quickly. Even when you do, he may not let go and forget what you said. Those with Asperger syndrome can have an excellent memory for dialogue, and their memory of what you said can sometimes seem unfairly selective. It is possible that, in particular, he will remember the negative things to the exclusion of anything else and perceive them to be a personal verbal attack on themselves.

Disclosure

Children with Asperger syndrome can sometimes have difficulty revealing what is bothering them. They can have tremendous problems at school and many have a history of severe bullying. This is rarely revealed to their parents or teachers, but is often bottled up inside. These feelings can then be projected on to something else. Often it is their parents who get the worst part of the deal. These children know that home is a safer place to express themselves than anywhere else and so can save up a whole day's worth of anxiety and let it out in a fit of anger when they get home.

In a similar way, this can apply to adults and can be observed when they are meeting with a professional person, where they can be incredibly well-mannered and polite throughout the duration of the meeting. In most circumstances, this is not a problem, but when the person is a doctor, psychologist or a counsellor, for instance, this can be quite misleading as this is not how they are usually.

One couple went for couples counselling because the husband, who has Asperger syndrome, refused to communicate with his wife and would become angry if she approached him about it. The couple did not realise at the time that Asperger syndrome was the problem. He behaved impeccably in the counselling room and his wife became very frustrated and angry. She felt as if she had been labelled as 'the baddie' by both her husband and the counsellor. She felt as though the counsellor thought she was exaggerating the problems. It was a very bad experience for her and the couple did not return to counselling.

How to make the right approach

If there is a particular issue or problem that needs to be sorted out, it will probably be up to you to choose the right time and place to discuss it with your partner. A time when you will not be interrupted and there will be no distractions is best, and the atmosphere between you needs to be as calm and stress-free as possible.

If you think about the problem carefully and attempt to remain as objective as possible, and do not use any exaggerations, it is more likely that a solution will be found. If the attempt fails, it may be because your partner is not in the right frame of mind or perhaps the timing is wrong. Often, though, it can be the choice of words and the way in which things are said that cause a breakdown in communication.

Here are a few strategies you could try that will hopefully make communication run more smoothly.

Giving complete messages

Giving complete messages is vital if you want your partner to fully understand what it is you are trying to tell him. Complete messages should contain at least four forms of disclosure: stating the facts, your thoughts, your feelings and what it is you need.

The facts should be based on something you have seen, heard, read or personally experienced. Your interpretation of the facts, though, is likely to be influenced by your own beliefs and opinions, but it is important to be honest about how you feel. Feelings can trigger some strong defensive reactions in both ourselves and others, sometimes leading to anger. Such anger is often used as a defence, especially when feeling sad and vulnerable and self esteem is running a bit low. It can be employed to disguise vulnerability.

The final stage in giving a complete message is to tell your partner exactly what you need. Although expressing feelings such as insecurity would immediately signal that maybe a hug is needed, this will not always happen when the communication is with a partner who has Asperger syndrome. He will not be able to guess what you want: you have to tell him.

Using complete messages

Using complete messages can take time and practice and it is a skill both you and your partner can learn. One couple I came into contact with had endless arguments about what appeared, on the surface, to be relatively trivial subjects. He described her as always angry and ready to 'attack' him; she was at her wits end and felt frustrated by the constant cycle they seemed to get caught up in. We discussed talking in complete messages and began to practise this skill and put it into operation.

One thing that they often fell out about was the way he would forget to give her a hug when he went to work. The tension would build up throughout breakfast. She would glare at him across the table; he had no idea what he had doing wrong but knew she was mad at him. This often resulted in him rushing out of the house as quickly as possible without so much as a goodbye, which left her feeling very rejected and vulnerable. Neither had discussed this pattern or ever said how it made them feel. We worked at putting this into a complete message and this resulted in the couple communicating as follows:

He: 'I can see by your face that you are mad at me, I think you are about to start shouting at me, I feel afraid because I do not know how to prevent it, I need to get away as quickly as possible.'

She: 'You keep forgetting to give me a hug before you go to work – I think you do it on purpose. It makes me feel very rejected and hurt. I need you to remember to hug me.'

From being able to communicate in complete messages both understood what the other wanted to say and they agreed to put a notice on the door to remind him to give her a hug. When the hug became a habit the notice was no longer needed. She had learnt not to disguise her feelings with anger and he had learnt that if he gave her a hug, she would be happy and he could enjoy his breakfast.

Always use the word 'I'

It is also important when you are explaining something to your partner, especially your feelings, always to remain in 'adult mode' – that is, always make use of the word 'I', not the word 'you', which can appear to be an accusation. Imagine being on the receiving end of the following – how would you feel?

- 'You have really upset me.'
- 'How could you be so thoughtless?'
- 'You really were so selfish tonight.'
- 'Why did you have to be so rude to my mother?'
- 'You think more about your precious (CD collection/magazines, etc.) than you do about me!

All these statements may seem quite justified at the time that they are said, but they would be interpreted by your partner as being critical and 'attacking' him. All sound far better if you rephrase them using the word 'I'.

- 'I feel quite upset by what was said earlier – maybe we could try to sort it out.'
- 'I felt that my feelings were not considered earlier on and this has left me feeling not cared for.'

- 'I felt my needs weren't acknowledged tonight and that has upset me.'
- 'Did my mother say something to upset you? I could not understand why you said ... to her.'
- 'I would like you to spend more time with me, I feel lonely sometimes.'

When partners interact, it is important that each takes responsibility for their own feelings and does not make assumptions about what the other is feeling. This is important to remember as it will give you a far better chance of getting your partner to listen and not interpret what is being said as being a critical attack on them, which could just make them withdraw or become defensive.

How to respond and not react

An important lesson to learn when developing communication skills is to respond, but not react. This can make the difference between a conversation between you running smoothly and reaching a satisfactory conclusion or rapidly escalating into a heated debate.

It is not always easy when you are feeling tired or frustrated to stop yourself from reacting to a situation or a statement made by your partner. However, the results of doing so are nearly always negative and achieve little, whereas responding maybe with a question and giving your partner time and the feeling that it is safe to reply can achieve a far more positive outcome. To react can often sound like you are blaming your partner for something, but to respond is to remain open and not accuse.

For example, one woman's husband accused her of not keeping the house very clean. Her immediate reaction was one of defence and attack, her reaction was, 'How dare you criticise me, if you do not like the way I keep the house then I suggest you do it yourself!' The consequence was an instant row.

Responding instead of reacting might first require a couple of deep breaths to help remain calm. This will also give a little time to think of an appropriate response. An appropriate response should be presented in the form of a question or using a complete message and the reaction above could be replaced with, 'You say I am not keeping the house clean. I think I work very hard and this is unjustified. I feel very hurt and need you to explain what exactly it is you are referring to.' The partner will now be aware of the effect his accusation has had on her and have the opportunity to be more precise and explain. In the case of this example, it turned out that she had forgotten to iron his shirt for work and he was feeling jealous about the extra time she was spending with the children.

Never assume

You should never assume that you know what your partner is thinking or that he knows what you are thinking. This can be especially problematic if you are a woman living with a man who has Asperger syndrome.

Most women can be very intuitive and pick up on an atmosphere and someone else's inner feelings quite quickly. They can often be far better at using and reading non-verbal language than most men. This strong intuition gives a woman an advantage over a man at interpreting non-verbal communication and, in most circumstances, this can work to a woman's benefit – unless, that is, she is living with a partner who has Asperger syndrome. Then, the non-verbal signals and body language sent out by her partner will not always accurately reflect what he is actually thinking or feeling. That this is so is evident from the poor eye contact that can be part of the non-verbal behaviour of people with Asperger syndrome, male or female. Evasive eye contact can give the impression that a person is lying. Often, though, in the case of people with Asperger syndrome, they are not lying, just poor communicators. It can also be that they smile or laugh at the wrong time and their partners are left thinking that they are making fun of them or not taking them seriously, when it is more likely to be a case that they do not know how to react. A smile can make someone happy, but, at the wrong time, it can appear very patronising. Many of the non-verbal reactions that adults with Asperger syndrome use have been learnt; they are not always automatic, and so have to be thought through.

You should never presume that your partner automatically knows or has picked up on what you are feeling. To expect a person with Asperger syndrome to know what someone is thinking, no matter how intimate they are, would be like expecting a blind person to guess what someone is holding in their hand without giving them any clues. Your partner cannot read minds and does not know instinctively from your expressions or body language what it is they are expected to do or say.

One way that your partner can be helped to understand what is expected of him is to use a written form of communication and this is described in the next section.

GETTING THE MESSAGE ACROSS

Writing things down

Tony Attwood[3] strongly recommends that it is simpler for each partner to write things down in letter or note form than to try and express verbally what each is trying to say or ask. This idea has certainly proved successful in my own experience when counselling couples when one of the partners has Asperger syndrome. It is a technique that I frequently use in the counselling room as it can offer great insight into what is really going on for both partners. One man with Asperger syndrome whom I interviewed was only able to communicate his deeper feelings through letter writing and he did this with profound literal accuracy and a great depth of feeling. They proved invaluable to his wife and compensated for what he never said. Letter writing gave him the time to think about what he wanted to say or what was bothering him.

For some couples writing things down, such as lists or reminders, works very well and can make giving instructions or directions for something far less complicated. One woman bought her husband a diary and he used it to write down important appointments, any arrangements he made with her and the children, or any jobs he had agreed to do on a particular day. It proved to be an absolute life saver once it became part of his daily routine to look in it.

Getting a response can be a problem when using letter writing, as an issue may require an answer or a response quite quickly. It may be that your partner will just read the note and that's it! The note goes into his pocket or a drawer and then he just forgets all about it. If nothing is mentioned, you may feel impatient and so demand an answer. This may produce a defensive reaction rather than an understanding response and suddenly the relationship is back to square one, leaving you feeling unheard and misunderstood. Maybe it could be arranged between you beforehand that if a letter is given, then an answer, or at least an acknowledgement, should be given within 24 hours, either in letter form or verbally.

Incentive, motivation and change

One of the reasons that your partner may ignore what you are saying to him or asking him to do is because he has not been given any valid reason to do otherwise. Writing letter after letter, list after list and pinning them up on noticeboards all over the house will make no difference at all unless he has an incentive to respond or do what you have asked of him. An incentive will increase his motivation, which will produce a change.

If he knows that if he does a certain thing it will make you happy and that, in return, you will, for example, go with him to the motor museum or give him some time out to pursue his favourite interest, there will be some incentive to respond. Sometimes, if he knows that doing something will mean that you will not get upset and his life will be easier, this alone can be enough of an incentive for him. If there is an incentive, and he understands what it is he needs to do, knowing that in return for his endeavours he will get something in return, he will be motivated. However, the payback for his actions has to be something that directly benefits him – not you, not the children, not the dog, only him.

One couple found an ideal compromise. He loved old cars and was quite an expert at restoring them. This he would do whenever he had any spare time, but at the expense of doing anything else. She, on the other hand, enjoyed the theatre, but he would not go with her, as he was always too occupied working on his cars, so they struck up a deal. Every other week she would spend a few hours with him, either helping him polish up the upholstery in one of his cars, or visiting a motor show and every other week he would go to the theatre with her. This worked well and enabled the couple to share something together.

Making use of the telephone and email

Letter writing may help your partner to say what is on his mind and sometimes email can be used to an even better effect than letter writing, as many people with Asperger syndrome enjoy spending time on the computer and the Internet, and you are already likely to have a collection of emails from him.

Partners with Asperger syndrome have also said that they find it easier to communicate on the telephone as they feel both safer and less confused in this situation. Talking on the telephone does not require them to use facial expression or eye contact, which can make them feel uneasy. Neither do they have to try to read others' expressions, so they are able to just concentrate on what is being said.

Talking with the lights turned down

Talking with the lights turned down can also reduce the confusion of mixed messages caused by misunderstanding non-verbal language and may feel more intimate than writing a letter.

Your partner may feel safer and more at ease when he cannot see your face and you cannot see his because he might just find it confusing to try to understand facial expressions *and* listen to your words and understand them at the same time. You should each try to keep your sides of the conversation equal in length and content and take turns to talk.

I normally recommend that couples try this while they are sitting together in the living room. I suggest that they turn off the television, turn down the lights, sit together, hold hands or whatever is most comfortable for them. It is wise to take the phone off the hook, make sure the children are in bed or out for the evening and then each take time to talk and listen. Listening is just as important as talking and you may have to be very patient and give your partner the time and space he needs to say what he wants to say. It is important to hear through what your partner is saying without jumping in making assumptions. If there is any opportunity to encourage him to talk about what is bothering him, it is important to make the most of it to reduce his anxiety and ensure your peace of mind.

Learning to listen

One of the reasons that your partner may not understand what you have said will be due to the way he may focus his attention on just a small part of what you are saying and will not appear to have heard the rest. When this happens repeat what was said and perhaps explain it in a different way. Check he has understood the meaning behind what was said by asking him to repeat it to you in his own words. One exercise that I found very useful when working with couples is the 'listening task' below.

Each partner takes turns in talking for two minutes about a completely neutral subject. During this time the other would have to listen and not interrupt. Afterwards they would repeat what they have heard to the partner who had spoken. Each partner would take turns each day to do this. As both become more equipped at listening the time could be extended, or more personal subjects could be talked about. Experiment with this exercise and see what works for you.

Dealing with one subject at a time

Too much information can cause sensory overload for your partner. This is why using a written form of communication or talking on the telephone can produce better results than a face-to-face conversation. Simultaneously interpreting non-verbal communication and understanding what is being said can require a lot of concentration from your partner. Also, using these other methods, the amount of information contained in each communication can be decreased, which will improve the chances of it being understood.

It is also important to deal with only one subject at a time. A statement such as the following example could cause utter chaos and produce only a negative reaction:

> *Well, what are you going to do about fixing the leak in the bathroom?*
> *Should we call a plumber? I have been asking you to do something*
> *for days – why do you always ignore me? You're just like your father*
> *– he never listened to a thing your mother said. I am sick of it. Well*
> *don't just stand there, shut the front door, I've just made a pot of tea.*

After such an onslaught, your partner may run the other way, freeze or react with anger. It is doubtful that he will either fix the tap or want a cup of tea. It is important, therefore, to remember to only ask one question about one subject at a time.

Summing up – the golden rules of communication

Here are the main points to remember when communicating with your partner:

- no ambiguous messages
- no double meanings
- use complete messages
- use the word 'I', not 'you'
- give an incentive
- never presume to know what he is thinking or feeling
- be clear, precise and straight to the point
- deal with one subject at a time
- give time and space for him to reply and tell you what his perspective on the situation is
- use any medium that helps to improve communication.

ANGER AND ASPERGER SYNDROME

Anger is an issue

Some women living with a partner who has Asperger syndrome have reported that their partners have a profound fear of confrontation and will do anything to avoid a display of anger directed at them. Those with the syndrome whom I have interviewed have all said that this is so, and it seems that this is especially the case when it is the male partner who has Asperger syndrome.

This fear manifests itself in the form of being unreasonably defensive, not speaking, leaving the room – anything rather than have their partner direct their anger at them. One woman's partner would disappear for days when she became angry with him. He reasoned that if he stayed away long enough, eventually she would have to calm down. The trouble was that, by the time he returned, she would be completely frantic after having contacted all the local hospitals, their family and friends, only to find out that he had spent the past couple of days looking at medieval church architecture.

A heightened sensitivity to anger

For men with Asperger syndrome, the fear of anger seems to be exaggerated completely out of proportion. It could be that you find yourself being accused of being angry when you are not. It is often that the partner with Asperger syndrome misreads the signals and thinks a particular look or tone of voice represents anger.

This can be very frustrating when you are trying to discuss a matter with your partner and before you know it, everything is out of proportion and a row is developing. You will need to learn to recognise this pattern and stop it before it develops, either by ending the conversation, changing the subject or agreeing to save it till later. In the counselling room I suggest that couples make rules beforehand and agree that they will bring the discussion to a quick end if it feels too uncomfortable.

One couple used a colour system to let each other know how they felt: green stood for 'OK', amber 'starting to feel unsure', and red meant 'I want to stop this now'. His wife would ask him what colour he felt: if he said red, for instance, then they would leave the subject until things felt calmer. It is completely useless for you to use anger as a means of expression or to get your point across. Some women reported trying to suppress their anger for this reason. This, though, can have a detrimental effect on both your mental and physical health.

Depression can be the result of anger turned inwards

Many of the women living with men with Asperger syndrome reported suffering from depression.

Some of them had probably realised that anger is a useless emotion in their relationship and so tried to suppress it. This suppressed anger can develop into depression and the long-term effects of this can be a deterioration in both the mental and physical health of the person involved.

It is important that ways of releasing anger are explored. Many women have tried different therapies, exercise programmes, counselling and outside support to help them vent their anger in a controlled and safe way.

Finding a positive channel for anger

The most effective and appropriate way for you to alleviate the effects of suppressed anger will depend on your individual circumstances – your age, lifestyle, financial situation and overall level of physical fitness.

If you are physically able, sports of any kind can be a marvellous outlet, whether it is gentle exercise – such as golf, yoga, Tai chi, swimming, walking – or more assertive sports – such as squash, running, badminton or aerobics. All these can help to release that stored-up aggression and energy in a positive way. One woman related how she had joined the local running club and ended up completing the London Marathon!

Other men and women I contacted relied on their religious faith to help get them through. They found that the support they received from their religious group or through prayer to be of tremendous value.

Some of the adults I spoke with had found individual counselling to be beneficial. It gave them time to talk about anxieties and express their anger to someone who could offer support and understand how they felt. They found this to be an excellent way of releasing frustrations. It is important when you are seeking counselling that the counsellor selected is aware of, and understands, the effects of Asperger syndrome on a relationship. Counselling can be sought through an agency or privately.

What about Asperger anger?

Anger can explode quite suddenly and seemingly for no reason in some individuals with Asperger syndrome. It can be something quite trivial that triggers their anger, and sometimes this can result in the nearest object to hand being broken. The suddenness and strength of the anger can be quite frightening to witness, especially when it is directed at you or your children, as the chances are that it will be completely irrational and unexpected.

It is important to try not to return this with your own anger (easier said than done), as your partner's anger will normally diffuse very quickly. Indeed, he will probably wonder what everyone is so upset about and could appear quite unaware what a painful and disturbing experience it was for you.

Some women reported instances of their partner's anger being channelled into road rage or directed at some innocent bystander and having tried to reason with him about the unfairness and irrationality of it. It can be very difficult to try and discuss your partner's anger with him. At times when he seems to have heard what has been said and change looks hopeful, this may be short-lived. Adults with Asperger syndrome can appear to go onto 'automatic pilot' when faced with particular situation and certain triggers are present.

For example, one woman's husband used to get extremely irate when anyone drove too close behind him and he would go to extreme and sometimes dangerous lengths to challenge the other driver's presence. He saw the other driver as the enemy and would become so focused on watching him in the mirror that he was in danger of not concentrating on the road ahead and causing an accident. This scared his wife and she had told him how she felt. Her partner, though, seemed unable to break this pattern and ignore the car behind him. In cases like this it can be a good idea to talk to a professional as the adult with Asperger syndrome is often more likely to listen to a third party than their partner. In this example the couple discussed it in counselling, and the woman's husband agreed that whenever this happened he would pull over when it was safe to do so and let the car behind pass.

Anger management in relationships where one partner has Asperger syndrome is certainly an area that needs more investigation. Programmes aimed at helping people with Asperger syndrome find ways to control their anger should eventually become available.

SEX AND ASPERGER SYNDROME

Loneliness in the bedroom

Some women living with a partner who has Asperger syndrome reported a complete lack of sexual intimacy in their relationship. In some cases, sexual intercourse had only occurred once or twice and then ceased altogether, leaving the female partner feeling very rejected, unloved and wondering what they had done wrong. Women with Asperger syndrome have also reported finding sexual intimacy difficult and not thinking of it as a necessary part of the relationship. So, it is probable that both men and women with Asperger syndrome experience sexual problems in their relationships.

It is important that you are aware that this is often not a reflection of a lack of love for you, but is more likely part of Asperger syndrome. Those with Asperger syndrome may not always require close physical or sexual contact with another person and would rather masturbate or abstain from sex totally. For some adults living with a partner with Asperger syndrome, the sexual side of the relationship is not very important to them and so they are more able to cope with a lack of it, while others may channel their sexual energy elsewhere.

Those who feel that sexual intimacy is very important to them do not cope with its absence very well and so this area of the relationship soon becomes one that breeds frustration and bitterness. Unless he is willing to try and sort something out about it and listen to what is being said, the situation will probably not change. Eventually you will have to make your own decisions as to whether or not the plusses in the relationship compensate for the loss of sexual intimacy.

There has been little research into and exploration of the sexual implications of Asperger syndrome, but hopefully in the future this will change and there will be more support and help on offer to couples.

Sometimes sex can become an obsession

It is not always the case that adults with Asperger syndrome do not have or want sex. For some, the sexual side of the relationship is not unlike that of any other couple and both parties report a happy and fulfilling sex life together.

In a few cases, however, it has been reported that the partner became obsessive in their endeavours to achieve perfection in their sexual role and would practise until they felt they had achieved the most perfect and rewarding sexual routine that they could. Some women reported that they were left feeling very used, as if they were being experimented on.

There is also the danger that once the 'perfect' routine has become established, it will not be changed. Restricted by this routine, sex can become regimented. Although they may be putting a lot of effort into pleasing their partner, the whole sexual act can come to feel like a process that follows a set order from beginning to end.

So, what happens if you are not satisfied by your sex life and want to try something else? An attempt to do something different or to change the routine could cause confusion and misunderstandings. Your partner could find this need to change very difficult and take it as a criticism of his lovemaking abilities. He may react negatively and you could end up feeling ignored and unheard, the self-esteem and confidence in both of you shattered.

Sex is a form of communication

Communication has been highlighted as problematic in relationships when one partner has Asperger syndrome, and as sex is also a form of communication, it is no exception. Sometimes the reason for sexual problems could be easily rectified if the partners were able to discuss their differences in clearer detail, and more important is that the adult without Asperger syndrome does not make any assumptions about their partner's behaviour. Things that might seem quite trivial to others may prove to be of great importance to the partner with Asperger syndrome.

For example, one partner with Asperger syndrome suddenly refused to have any sexual contact with his wife. He became very unresponsive and unaffectionate. This had lasted for over twelve months when eventually the couple came for counselling. Time and patience were given while the partner with Asperger syndrome was allowed to explore his feelings and reasons for not having sex. He talked about his toiletries, and in particular his toothbrush. He had a certain way of leaving his razor, shaving foam and toothbrush in a particular order on the shelf behind the sink every morning. Every evening when he came to brush his teeth, he found his wife had placed his brush into a cup with everyone else's. This annoyed him immensely and by the time he got into bed he was too angry to even touch his wife. After discussing this further, his wife was able to understand how important it was to him and agreed that she would leave the toothbrush where it was. Their love life slowly returned to normal.

Where does the information about sex come from?

Just as most adults with Asperger syndrome learn how to socialise and interact from books or television programmes, this can also be the case for sexual activities. What they say and do in bed can depend on what they have read or seen on television. Women have reported their partners coming out with some most unusual statements in the middle of sex and often being shocked by what can sometimes seem quite crude remarks that are completely out of character.

Others will ask rather strange, clinical questions that can make sex feel like a biological experiment.

Often, these statements or questions come from something your partner has watched on television, read in a magazine or overheard at work. It is wise to have an idea where your partner gets his information from as this can affect how he regards his role and your role in your sexual relationship. If he is reading pornographic magazines, visits sites on the Internet or is receiving information from a biased source, he may be led to believe that behaviour which you find quite unacceptable is appropriate.

There are plenty of good and reliable reading materials around and some books offer a visual guide that may make it easier for your partner. If either of you finds it hard to talk about sex, then you could consider going to counselling together or seeking the help of a psycho-sexual therapist.

For most relationships, it is important to know that sex is something very special, shared between the two of you, and not just a performance or simply a means to an end.

Getting it right from the start

If your relationship is quite a new one, then it is crucial that both of you start as you mean to go on. It is helpful if you can be patient with your partner and try to tell him in a precise and clear way what you want in bed and what you are prepared to give. If your relationship is well established, it can be harder to change things, but not impossible.

It is important when communicating about sex not to be ambiguous and not to give double messages. Your partner cannot read your mind – he does not know what you want or do not want unless you tell him. Whether or not your relationship is a new one, stress to your partner that you will not want the same things every time, that your needs will change. Reassure him that you will tell him if there is something you do not want, so he will know if he is doing something wrong. Perhaps explain a woman's sexual cycle, pointing out that at certain times of the month you may be more responsive than others. Be sure he knows your different reactions to him are not because of something he has done wrong, but that this is just the way most women are and that needs and sexual appetites change.

It is important that both of you feel comfortable about what you are doing. No one in a sexual relationship should have to do anything they feel uncomfortable with. As your partner may have more difficulty with discussing sexual issues, it is helpful to check that he is happy with the lovemaking and what is being shared together.

Be positive

When you discuss sex with your partner, you should do so in a sensitive way, taking care not to sound critical. Positive and constructive examples should be given of how sex can be enjoyed more together, so that he knows exactly what you want. If possible, these should be explained in a visual way. You should try to find a time when you will not be disturbed and the atmosphere is calm and relaxed. You should also choose your words carefully and be tactful, suggesting rather than demanding, and respect each other's freedom of choice. Follow the golden rules for communication discussed earlier.

Infidelity and Asperger syndrome

In most cases, women reported that they had complete trust in their partner's fidelity to them, and for many this is a very positive aspect of their relationship. In Debbie Then's[15] book, she reported that 50 percent of men in the general population are likely to stray, yet in 80 percent of the couples I contacted, the women were totally convinced that their husbands were faithful and would remain that way. The security this creates is a huge boon in any relationship and can mean that women tolerate the more negative effects of Asperger syndrome in their relationships.

It needs to be said, however, that for those rare men with Asperger syndrome who are unfaithful, this can become a pattern that is very hard to change.

PARENTING

Mainly for women

This section has been written for women who are living with a male partner who has Asperger syndrome. Women with the syndrome to whom I have spoken did not have any children, so I cannot speak with any authority on how relationships between men who have a female partner with the syndrome are affected by pregnancy and the arrival of children. I would like, however, to suggest that you read Liane Holliday Willey's book, *Pretending to be Normal*,[16] which gives us a wonderful insight into being a wife and a mother when you have Asperger syndrome. It is certainly worth a read, especially if you are a man and you suspect or know that your female partner has Asperger syndrome.

Pregnancy

Pregnancy, childbirth and parenting can be especially problematic in a relationship when your partner has Asperger syndrome.

Pregnancy is a time when bonding is very important, but for some women I spoke to it was quite a lonely time and their partner was very reluctant to have any sexual contact with them, leaving them feeling unwanted and undesirable. For some men with Asperger syndrome this can be because they fear that they will do some harm to their unborn child and so they feel they should not maintain sexual intimacy during this time. This fear may come from mixed messages about pregnancy received in childhood and adolescence.

It is important to involve your partner as much as possible with the pregnancy and explain exactly what is happening physically, using visual means if possible. You need to encourage him to ask questions and make him feel very much a part of the whole pregnancy.

Giving birth

It has been reported that some fathers-to-be did not want to be present at the birth of their child. One woman relayed how her partner quite simply did not turn up at the hospital, which caused her to feel very alone at a time that should be one of sharing.

Unpredictable and stressful social situations can be quite traumatic for someone with Asperger syndrome, and one of the reasons the birth of their child may be avoided is because they may not have any idea what their role will be and what will be expected of them. If possible, watch a video on childbirth together so that your partner knows exactly what it will be like and what you want him to do.

It is very difficult at a time like this for you to have to worry about your partner – you will probably feel that he should be worrying about you rather than the other way round. This can leave some women feeling cheated out of what should be a loving, caring, shared experience.

If possible (usually it is positively encouraged), both of you should arrange to go along together to antenatal classes and visit the labour and maternity wards at the hospital where you are planning to have your baby to meet one or more of the midwives or hospital staff. This will help make the forthcoming birthplace feel more familiar and less threatening for your partner. Encourage him to ask questions and help him to understand what a very necessary and important part of the whole birth experience he is.

Life after birth

Looking after a baby seems, in most cases where the father has Asperger syndrome, to have been left entirely up to the mother as he takes on the role of a distant observer. Some women have not found this to be a problem if, as with the financial side of the relationship, they prefer to be in control of the situation and be the main decision maker. Other women, however, found this a desperately lonely time and felt at times that they were surviving on the same level as a one-parent family, with little or no practical or emotional support from their partner.

It needs to be remembered that this scenario can be played out in any relationship. Not all men, whether they have Asperger syndrome or not, want to participate in looking after a baby. They may find this stage of child development especially difficult, and for men it can even be quite frightening. What is probably different about the situation when the father has Asperger syndrome is that they can display a lack of empathy towards their partner and do not appear to appreciate how much hard work emotionally and physically looking after a new baby can be. If you are blessed with an understanding doctor, or know of another professional that understands Asperger syndrome, ask if he or she could talk to your partner. Your partner may be able to tell them what is bothering him and how he feels about the baby and they may be able to offer him some advice or extra information. Try all avenues open to you and if your partner is still unable to offer you any consideration or appreciation, then you may find that you have to find this emotional support elsewhere.

Negotiate the rules

As the children grow, your partner may have problems both in making himself understood and in being understood by his children. It is common in people with Asperger syndrome not to discriminate between ages and it could be particularly difficult for your partner to talk to the children as children and be aware of what levels of development and maturity they have reached. His expectations of his children's capabilities may be set a lot higher than they are actually capable of achieving, and this can cause confusion for all concerned.

Your partner may not know or understand what he is expected to do or say to the children. For example, one mother described how her nine year old son had brought home his report for his parents to read. His father read through the report quite quickly and then without a word to his son about how well he had done, wrote a lengthy reply to the headmaster. He complained that he was unable to read the

English teacher's comments and asked how could she possibly teach his son when her handwriting was illegible. What he had not done in all this was to tell his son what an excellent school report he had brought home, he could only focus on the English teacher's handwriting. His wife had tried to explain to him that he was missing the point, but it was not until he had written and sent in his letter that he could tell his son it was a good report.

You will often need to state the obvious and always give very clear and precise messages, so that he understands what he is supposed to do or say. It is very important that you negotiate the rules between yourselves and both try to stick to them.

If you have a problem trying to negotiate rules and boundaries and if there is a problem enforcing these rules, then you could try talking it over with a third party, such as a counsellor or teacher. Making use of noticeboards, lists or diaries is also useful. One woman had lists all over the house, even in the bathroom, giving clear instructions on hanging up the towels, putting the seat down on the toilet (so the youngest did not fall down into the bowl) and flushing the toilet. You should experiment with whatever methods work best in your household. If it turns out to be a useful and helpful strategy, then it should be put into practice on a daily basis. Children need a consistent, loving and caring upbringing, and it is you who might find yourself being left with most of the responsibility for seeing that they are provided with this.

Teenage terrors – the Asperger nightmare

Parenting may have been fairly straightforward while the children were young enough to obey commands and rules without arguing about them. All this can change when they hit adolescence, start bringing friends home and answering back.

Your partner probably never understood his own adolescence, so it is very unlikely that he will understand it in his own children. He may find their disruptive routines, changeable timetables, faddy eating habits, unpredictable moods, answering back and constant demand for lifts an Asperger nightmare and will certainly suffer from teenage terrors. It could feel like there is an additional teenager in the house and you may wonder who is the harder work – the children or him.

One woman's husband used to spend his time trying to get his daughter to be more tidy. He went as far as putting his daughter's homework in with the rubbish because she had left it on the kitchen table. He felt this was quite justified and would not apologise for his actions. The whole family was in an uproar and it was his wife who had to write a letter to the school and try to smooth things over. You will have to be the mediator, negotiator, referee, rule-maker, wiper up of tears, confidante – in other words, all things to all people.

If your children know about Asperger syndrome, you could ask them to be more sensitive and try to understand why there are some things that their father does not get right or understand. It should be explained to them that things that cause their father stress and frustration should be avoided. House rules need to be negotiated for the whole family.

You will need all the help you can get. As you will be the one giving out all the emotional energy, you must be aware of your own needs at this time – otherwise, you will be left feeling completely drained and very alone. You should try to make some time for yourself and put your needs first at times, whether this takes the form of a visit to the hairdressers, a night out with friends or a hobby that gets you out of the house. It is vital that you have time and space that is completely separate from your partner and the children where you can just unwind and be yourself, free from any demands.

MONEY MATTERS

Sorting out the finances

In most cases, the couples I contacted reported that it was the partner who did not have Asperger syndrome who looked after the financial side of things in the relationship and, largely, this seemed to work quite well. Problems can arise if your partner has an expensive special interest, such as collecting rare old coins. It is important that you are aware of what is happening to the finances, especially if money is not abundant. In a few cases where the partner without Asperger syndrome was not allowed any control of the money matters at all, there were massive debts.

Whether or not poor money management skills are a consequence of Asperger syndrome is impossible to say as I have also talked to women who say their husbands are excellent at dealing with the finances. It is often found in adults with Asperger syndrome that there is an inclination towards extremes, shown by either being very capable at doing a particular task or by finding it very difficult. This area has not been studied sufficiently and, certainly, financial problems can occur in any relationship, whether one of the partners has Asperger syndrome or not. The difference Asperger syndrome makes in a relationship is that it introduces an extra level of difficulty when trying to discuss financial problems. It can be hard to get your partner to talk about monetary matters and establish the rules and boundaries.

Knowing what is being spent

It is important that you know what is happening on the financial front. If at all possible, either deal with the finances yourself or at least maintain some form of independence. This is not so difficult to do today as it was a few decades ago as many women now control their own finances. As mentioned earlier, telling others is not high on the list of priorities for people with Asperger syndrome, so it could be the case that you will be the last to know about any financial problems that have been building up. This is probably because your partner is frightened of telling you what is happening and the reaction it might provoke. This is especially likely to be the case when the money is being spent on his special interest.

SPECIAL INTERESTS

It can be a bonus

Most of the adults I contacted said that their partners had a special interest, and most said they did not find it particularly problematic in the relationship, when compared to other areas, such as communication. In fact, some said that their partner's special interest was a bonus! Many were happy that their partner had something to interest them and keep them busy. One woman remarked that at least he was not chasing other women or 'living in the pub'.

Your partner's special interest is likely to be a solitary pursuit, such as collecting, exploring old churches or running. Life with someone who has Asperger syndrome may involve feeling similar to a 'golf widow' or widower. The special interest may also be linked to his field of work, perhaps in engineering or computers. Simon Baron-Cohen[6] found that, statistically, engineering occupations featured more predominantly in families in which Asperger syndrome was present.

Some of the special interests reported were a little unusual, even quite bizarre. One woman said that her husband purchased copies of every hi-fi magazine he could lay his hands on, and had been doing so for most of his life. The problem was that he would not throw any of them away. The collection had become so large that she was unable to get into their spare room, as it was literally full from floor to ceiling with magazines. Eventually there was no longer any room for anything else in their home, so they were looking for a bigger house. For most couples, the partner's special interest becomes a way of life. As long as it does not run the family into debt, it is tolerated and can be a very good talking point.

If obsessions do become a problem financially, it is important that this is dealt with in its earliest stages and not allowed to escalate. If it is possible for you to take charge of the finances, then this is often the best solution. Those who have managed to do this have found it a tremendous relief as then neither partner has to worry about what is happening to the money.

When a special interest is unacceptable

Although it appears to be quite rare in cases of Asperger syndrome, sometimes the partner's special interest is something that the other partner feels is totally unacceptable. It may be something that is counter to what would normally be permissible within a close relationship and then both partners need to do something about it. For instance, if he is obsessed with sex, pornography (possibly spending time seeking it on the Internet) or other women or men in a sexual way and has extramarital affairs, the other partner has the same rights as anyone else in a relationship when its boundaries are being crossed. If they find pornography offensive or are concerned that this is not setting a good example to the children, then they have the right to act and either end the relationship or demand that things change.

If your partner will not change and is also aware that his behaviour is unacceptable to you, then you have to make a choice: do or don't you want the relationship to continue?

Sharing interests

Some couples I spoke to shared similar interests – many reported that they enjoyed going to the theatre together, listening to music or seeing films at the cinema, for example. Others shared the same religious beliefs and their faith was very important to them. As long as you are prepared to do things your partner's way and able to relate to the area of interest, then this can be an excellent way for you to feel closer to each other and share things together. Also, if the interest is something new to you, there is the bonus that you will become an expert on something that you previously knew little or nothing about.

ROUTINES

Never-ending routines

Some adults with Asperger syndrome have some very rigid routines that they feel very strongly have to be followed through in the same order every time. It may be, for example, the 'getting ready for work' routine, the 'daily cleansing' routine, the 'cleaning the house' routine or the 'eating at the table' routine. Once a routine becomes established, it can soon become fixed, narrow and repetitive.

One woman described a life that had become a regimented nightmare, that revolved around the clock. Getting up, meal times and going to bed: her whole life was organised and controlled. How had it become this way? It appeared that when they first married, she had tried very hard to please him and had allowed him the control of the daily running of the house. She did not realise that once these routines became fixed she would be unlikely to get him to change them. It is very important not to allow strict routines to develop in the relationship, as once established, trying to change these routines could cause a lot of stress and anxiety for both of you.

When routines are a problem

If family life is totally regimented by routines the whole family may feel very controlled and life can feel as though nothing is ever spontaneous or fun.

If your relationship is relatively new, then you should endeavour to start as you mean to go on. Thus, if there is something your partner is doing that you really cannot stand, then try to stop it before it develops into a set pattern.

If the routine is already established, however, it can be very difficult or even sometimes impossible to change completely. Small changes are sometimes possible if the partner without Asperger syndrome is willing to stand her ground. For example, one woman's husband insisted that no-one was allowed to speak while they sat at the dinner table: meals had to be in absolute silence. Meal times for her and the children became very stressful and not an enjoyable experience. She told him unless he was more lenient they would all eat at separate times. This did not work, so she told him that in future he would have to get his own dinner. He then agreed to compromise and it was decided that they would not talk while eating but could talk before, after or in between courses. It was a small compromise and she had to be very firm and stand by her threat, but it achieved a change and helped alleviate some of the pressure.

Another way that can prove helpful in tolerating routines is to look for the positive. One woman's partner was obsessive about rubbish and would spend valuable time sorting out the household rubbish into bag after bag after bag. This routine drove her to distraction, yet when he went away on business, she found herself following the same routine. In doing so, she saw some logic in it. Since then, her partner's habit has no longer irritated her and at least she has the reassurance that he would never dream of forgetting to put the rubbish out for collection.

Routines can be useful

Most women I contacted talked about their partner's routines in favourable terms. Some said it was a relief that they never had to check the house was locked up at night and always knew the bath would be clean. One woman's partner always did his own ironing so that he could do it his way, which she was definitely very happy about.

A perfect job

Adults with Asperger syndrome can be very dependable and, if given something to do, as long as they want to do it, they will do it no matter what. They will complete the job and it will be done to perfection. It may take them a while – and you will have to be patient as he will not take short cuts or 'make do' – but the result will be worth it.

Different people with Asperger syndrome will be gifted in different ways. One woman described how her partner mapped out all her routes for her and, even though she had to sit with him for ages while he described every landmark on the way, she knew she would not get lost and would be grateful later for the comfort of knowing exactly where she was going.

SOCIALISING SOLUTIONS

Social problems

Many women told me about problems that occurred in social situations that made life very difficult at times. Sometimes your partner will do anything to avoid such events. Having problems with knowing how to interact socially with others is one of the core traits of Asperger syndrome, so it is inevitable that, some way or another, this area is going to be a challenge for your relationship. The exact problems, though, will vary from couple to couple, so the degree of disruption and inconvenience they cause will also vary.

The introvert

Most adults with Asperger syndrome seem to either display introvert or extrovert traits; the majority, however, appear to be quite introvert by nature. Introverts will go to any lengths to avoid social situations. For example, some partners quite simply refuse to socialise at all – some not coming home from work when they know that some event has been arranged or, if they do attend, they may fall asleep or be so rude to other people that their partner may wish they had not come. Some women have found themselves getting a taxi home as their partners have left them alone at a social gathering, disappearing altogether without any prior warning.

The extrovert

As well as the partners who avoid social situations, there are a few who go to the other extreme and behave in an extrovert way, especially if they have had a drink. They can become quite loud and overpowering, often making jokes that no one understands and can cause a lot of embarrassment for the partners who do not have Asperger syndrome. It may appear that their behaviour is reverting to that of adolescence and they are unaware of how they appear to others. Alternatively, they may start talking about their favourite hobby and some poor unsuspecting person becomes trapped in a one-way conversation (this can apply to both introverts and extroverts). The partner, meanwhile, will be totally unaware that he has been talking for too long and will not pick up the signals that he has overstayed his welcome.

Getting on better with the other sex

If your partner is male, then he may have a highly developed feminine side and so will often appear to get on better with women than men. This may be because he was bullied at school by other boys. Sadly, this happens to many boys with Asperger syndrome. He may find women are more tolerant of his lack of confidence and conversational topics, and he would have learnt quickly that he is more likely to be accepted by females than males.

Interestingly, I found that this was also the case for the women with the syndrome whom I contacted, but in reverse, as they showed a preference for male friends. A woman with Asperger syndrome described to me the difficulty she had in conversing with women. She said she found most women quite boring! Her topic of conversation with other women was quite restricted; she did not have children and had no desire to talk about her husband beyond to say what he did as a job and the fact he collected the *Radio Times*. She could, however, talk about nail varnish or her collection of hundreds of pairs of shoes. She had figured out that if she wanted to end a conversation with someone, she would simply go into great detail about the manufacture of toilet cleaner, as she said this never failed to help her escape from a situation she did not want to be in. It is possible that one of the reasons females with Asperger syndrome find that males are easier to get on with is because they make fewer emotional demands on them.

Inappropriate flirting

Sometimes those with Asperger syndrome can become quite fixed on one particular person, say at a party. If this person is of the opposite sex, this can create mixed messages. Your partner may stand too close to them or disclose too much information for just a casual chat. This situation can cause problems for other partners as it can look like blatant and inappropriate flirting. Unless you recognise what is happening quite quickly and tactfully interrupt and lead your partner away, it can cause upset and misunderstandings for all those involved.

Literal interpretation

Taking things literally and not understanding jokes and sarcasm can make socialising a nightmare for someone with Asperger syndrome. The women I have contacted in the course of my research have given accounts of some very awkward situations that have arisen because of their partner's misinterpretation of what someone has said or not knowing when something is a joke. For instance, one woman described a time at a party when her partner was asked jokingly, 'where he was coming from'. This completely confused him, and when he answered, very seriously, that he had just come from the toilet, everyone laughed. Her husband did not understand what he had said that was so funny. Likewise, not realising that honesty is not always the best policy when asked to give an opinion can cause problems. Those with Asperger syndrome will inevitably give a very honest answer, often causing offence.

Exaggerations

Exaggerations form part of our daily communication and we are often not aware we are even doing it. For example, we may say it rained for weeks when in fact it only rained for a couple of days, or we may say a journey took us all day, when it took only three hours. We accept these exaggerations, and know that the queue for the checkout was not miles long, and that there were not hundreds of people waiting for the bus.

The adult with Asperger syndrome may not know you are exaggerating and it is important that you tell your partner things as they really are. If you do not, you may find yourself being frequently corrected by him in public, or if he was not there with you he may take what you are saying very seriously. One woman had complained to her partner that her nail varnish took hours to dry and he discussed this with the receptionist at work, seriously convinced that his wife had told him the truth. The receptionist was unable to tell him that this was not normally the case and was probably left thinking that the whole conversation was rather bizarre.

Your partner will not understand exaggerations and to avoid embarrassment for both of you, you will need to be aware that you are saying is based on facts.

Not recognising the dangers

Another problem that was described by some of the women I spoke to was their partner's difficulty in recognising potentially dangerous situations. This may be due to not reading the signals, or because their partner has become focused on one particular thing. A situation described to me by one woman took place in the car park of a well known drive-in burger restaurant. Her husband noticed a group of rather rowdy men in a car throw all their empty cartons onto the car park. He got out of his car, walked over to their car, picked up their rubbish and chucked it back through their car window with the comment that he believed it to be theirs. He brushed his hands together and walked back to his car, got back in and drove away, luckily before they were able to react and get to him.

It may seem that the partner is being very brave and standing up for his beliefs, but it is more likely that he does not recognise the potential danger that he is putting both himself and his family into.

Difficulty transferring information

Often those with Asperger syndrome do not have the ability to transfer information from one situation to another. It is possible for your partner to learn that it is impolite to make comments on what a person is wearing, even if it really does not suit them, but what about when you want your partner's real opinion about something important? He will probably just agree with whatever is being said and leave you to make the decisions alone rather than run the risk of saying the wrong thing. This example can sound quite trivial, but, in fact, it is things like this that cause tension between you. You will feel that you are left with all the responsibility and that you do not know if your partner agrees with you or not. If you tell your partner that you will not get angry or upset if he tells you the truth about something, it is vital that you see this promise through, whatever the answer. If you do not do this, your partner will remember your reaction and probably be very reluctant to tell the truth again.

Thinking ahead

Unless your partner refuses to socialise under any circumstances, there is nothing to say that he cannot be helped to get through the social situations that are causing problems. You will, over time, probably develop a sixth sense for when you need to intervene to save a situation. You may, for example, notice that your partner has been talking for too long to a poor, but polite, guest, who is slowly learning all there is to know about your partner's pet subject. If you are planning to eat out, you can check in advance that the restaurant passes the 'Asperger test' – that is, it is very clean and has a selection of food that you both enjoy. Thinking ahead is always a useful strategy – prevention rather than cure.

If you know in advance that you are going to be in the company of people who are sensitive to particular issues or hold very strong beliefs or opinions, talk to your partner first and explain the subjects which are taboo and would be best left alone. Your partner often does not realise that sometimes his sense of humour or honesty can be very upsetting for someone else. The sense of humour of an adult with Asperger syndrome can often be very adolescent in nature. Sometimes jokes are repetitive and therefore become irritating rather than funny. One man I spoke to who had Asperger syndrome always made rhymes out of people's names which were not always complimentary: I never asked what his rhyme was for my name!

Many difficult situations have been described to me over the years. One woman described how her husband made jokes about bodybags while visiting her mother in the hospital, where she had just had a major operation. Another woman explained her utter disbelief when her husband told one of their friends that she smelled. No-one knew what to say and all just stood in complete silence. Luckily his wife tried to brush it aside by telling her friend not to worry because he says that to her all the time and it just meant that they must be wearing the same perfume. With that, she grabbed her husband by the arm and marched him off.

Situations like this can be embarrassing and sometimes very hurtful for others. In time you will become more aware of certain tricky situations and the areas of conversation to avoid. You will be able to brief your partner on what not to say, and what subjects not to mention such as religion, politics or homosexuality, to name a few.

A single focus

A feature of Asperger syndrome is that of becoming quite stuck and focused on one particular object or subject. One woman described how her husband always seemed to become obsessed with the seating arrangements whenever they went out for a meal. He saw it as his duty to make certain everyone sat in the order he found appropriate, which normally placed him as far away from the children as possible. He would achieve this even if it involved the entire family having to get up and move around the table. At times like this his wife decided it was easier to let him just get on with it rather than cause a fuss in a public place. He would only have argued that he was only trying to look after everyone and that he was acting in their best interest.

Always doing their best

It can be helpful to allocate something useful for your partner to do on social occasions. If you are having a party, you can ask your partner to take care of the drinks, the food or, better still, the music. It can be guaranteed that your partner will soon have the CDs completely organised and, although everyone will have to spend the entire evening listening to his choice of music, it will be sorted out and you will not have to worry about it.

A word of warning, though: think carefully about the tasks that you give to your partner as he will take them very seriously and not stop until the mission is completed. One woman told me about a fireworks display that the entire family, including aunts and uncles, went to one bonfire night. It was taking place in the grounds of an old castle. She asked her husband, who was more familiar with the layout of the castle grounds than she was, if he could find the best possible place for them to stand to see the fireworks. He certainly found the best place, but the effort it took to get there was quite traumatising, climbing over rocks and down slippery slopes all at a rate of knots, with her husband rushing ahead like a squadron leader, ordering everyone around. By the time the family got there, no one was in the right frame of mind to enjoy the display – two family members had walked off and the poor wife was a complete nervous wreck.

Your partner's determination to complete a task can, therefore, be a bonus, but only if it is channelled in the right direction.

The deserter

If, while entertaining, your partner wants to go to another room and look through his favourite magazines or go for a walk or to bed, does it really matter? He has not really deserted or abandoned you and he will have given as much time as he can manage. Maybe socialising is not his thing and it probably was not his choice to be in this social situation in the first place.

If friends know that he has Asperger syndrome, then they will understand that socialising is difficult for him. If friends do not know, then they can be told that your partner is very tired or feeling unwell.

Many women have become experts at making excuses for their partners and covering up for them. Unfortunately, however, your partner may not appreciate how hard you try to smooth things over for him, so sometimes it may seem that all your efforts are completely unreciprocated. He may not show any empathy for the sacrifices that you have made for him, which can make it hard to bear. Is this part of Asperger syndrome or is your partner just being selfish? The next section answers this question.

EMPATHY AND RECIPROCITY

Lack of empathy

Empathy is the ability to put yourself in someone else's shoes. Having a lack of empathy is one of the aspects of Asperger syndrome that partners find hardest to deal with. This problem is intensified because not empathising means that partners are unlikely to be appreciated for all the effort, time and self-sacrifice they have to put into the relationship because of the presence of the syndrome.

Your partner is unlikely to be upset because he has upset you, but will be if your reaction to something affects his routine or interferes with the way he is treated. It is easier for both of you if you know that this lack of empathy and appreciation for your efforts is not him being intentionally hurtful. Your partner is not holding anything back – he is probably unaware of what he should do or feel grateful for. Indeed, he is unlikely to have any idea what it is that you are getting so upset and stressed about.

Adults with Asperger syndrome are just being themselves and doing things in their own way. They do not have any particular problems with the way they are – they are doing what they want in the way they want to do it. They may see their partner as being the one with the problem, the one who complains and moans all the time. Because of their lack of empathy, they may not be able to see that the problem their partner has stems from something to do with their behaviour.

Asperger syndrome or just being selfish?

The behaviour of those with Asperger syndrome can appear very selfish, but this is part and parcel of the disorder and they are probably not even aware that what they are doing is sometimes very one-sided. Your partner may expect his daily routine to remain unchanged or for you to be interested and listen patiently when he is trying to tell you something about his special interest. He may also insist that you do certain things the way he wants them to be done.

It sounds like the ultimate in selfishness that the only needs he is bothered about are his own, but, in fact, it is simply that he is unaware of how some things he does come across to others. His behaviour is a consequence of Asperger syndrome, which means he has difficulty conceptualising how his partner feels and does not have the ability to put himself in someone else's shoes. This does not mean that he does not care or feel concern for his partner, but that he is not able to imagine what his partner is feeling.

Reciprocity means to feel or give in return for the same. Most relationships depend on reciprocity to make them work – there has to be give and take. Some women I contacted felt that they gave and their partners took.

However, no amount of nagging, emotional blackmail or ultimatums will make any difference. These will just put your partner under tremendous pressure, because he will not know how to show or express this thing you call empathy.

For the relationship to continue less stressfully, you need to maintain a realistic view of the situation and not strive for the impossible. Your partner cannot give you something he does not have, but he can protect you, care, show concern and give comfort if he is made aware that this is what is required of him.

Externalising the blame

One of the ways in which some women coped in such a non-reciprocal relationship was by externalising all their partner's negative traits, blaming them on Asperger syndrome. Many of the women said that once they had a diagnosis or were certain that their partner had the syndrome, they developed a wonderful ability to attribute all their partner's lack of empathy and reciprocity to the syndrome, which then became the scapegoat. They blamed Asperger syndrome as if it were a third party and then could live with their partners' behaviour.

Externalisation of blame is not unusual – it is a way of dealing with the flaws our loved ones have. Often when things go wrong for people, such as failing at a task, they blame all manner of things, from lack of time to the weather. The fact, then, that so many women blame Asperger syndrome for everything negative about their partner is not so unusual. It is, in fact, a brilliant strategy and it really works. Remember, though, that there are many things your partner can make choices about, just like anyone else.

ASPERGER SYNDROME CANNOT BE BLAMED FOR EVERYTHING

Just because your partner has Asperger syndrome does not mean that he has no choice but to do what he does in all areas of his life. It is not an excuse to be violent, aggressive or a control freak; it is not an excuse to gamble, nor is it an excuse to be unfaithful. There are many rules and boundaries within any relationship that have to be respected and in no way should anyone tolerate anything that they feel puts them or their children in danger or causes them extreme stress and heartbreak.

In all close relationships, whether Asperger syndrome is present or not, each partner has to decide what they are and are not prepared to tolerate. Certainly, if someone with Asperger syndrome is capable of forming an intimate relationship, they should also be quite capable of knowing that there are some types of behaviour that are totally unacceptable and inappropriate, and top of the list is domestic violence.

Domestic violence

Having Asperger syndrome is not an excuse to be physically violent or aggressive towards you or your children and should not be tolerated in any circumstances. Having the syndrome does not mean that your partner is more likely to be violent or aggressive – in fact, evidence from the women I have contacted suggests that physical violence appears to be quite uncommon.

Anger seems to be quite short-lived as well and can make its appearance in the form of a sudden outburst. There can be a build-up of daily hassles and then something seemingly irrelevant triggers explosive anger. This can be quite out of character and frightening. Some women have said that their partner will throw or break the nearest object to hand. Usually it is only the object that gets physically damaged, but what about the damage this can do to their partner's emotional well-being?

Anger without a cause

What follows will not apply to all adults with Asperger syndrome as not all of them have sudden bursts of anger. If your partner is one of those who does, you may be left wondering what you said or did to cause it, as this reaction can seem to come out of the blue and is often over something seemingly trivial.

Asperger anger seems to be sharp and very short-lived, so it will disperse as quickly as it appeared. Afterwards, your partner will be fine again and you will often be left wondering why he was so upset. You will feel wounded, attacked and probably in a flood of tears, while your partner will not understand what is wrong and may expect you to recover as quickly as he has. He will just want to get on with his day and for you to carry on as before and not disrupt any plans. It is you who will be left to deal with the aftermath alone.

After an argument

After an argument, it is helpful to have someone you can talk to who understands how you feel – maybe someone in the family or, even better, someone else who has a partner with Asperger syndrome. Talking is therapeutic, which is why counselling can be so useful. Maybe when things have calmed down, you can discuss the incident with your partner using the golden rules of Asperger syndrome communication mentioned earlier.

One couple found that letter writing worked best for them if she felt hurt or upset by something he had done or said. She would write him a letter and leave it somewhere for him find it. This allowed him to sit quietly and read what she had written. He would then email her from work or write her a note back. This way both could say what they wanted without being interrupted. This way worked for them but another way may work for you. Decide, between you, at a time when you are both feeling close which way would feel most comfortable for you both.

Displaced anger

Sometimes it turns out that the angry outburst is not about you at all, which explains why it seems to come from nowhere and the feeling that it does not relate to anything you were talking about or doing at the time. One woman described just such an incident. She had asked her husband to pick up a paper on the way home from work. When he arrived home and had forgotten the paper, she said in a half humorous way that he could not be depended on for anything and she would not ask him again. He 'went up in the air like a rocket', picked up a chair and broke it. The children ran into the room as they were so concerned, and, without speaking, he stormed out of the house. She just stood there amazed. She felt she was the one who should have been angry and was very upset by the whole episode. Her husband returned home later, but would not discuss the incident. It was only the next day, when she spoke to a friend who worked with him, that she discovered he had had a really bad day at work. He had complained that some of the other men were not pulling their weight and spent more time reading the paper than doing their work.

It is clear from this that he had contained his anger at work, ignoring it when workmates had made some pretty cruel remarks to him, but had internalised the negative effect of the whole episode. The anger he unleashed as a reaction to what his wife said belonged with the men at work, but she got the whole lot, and all because he thought she was running him down. He was, sadly, unable to detach one situation from another and placed her in the same category as the men back on the shop floor.

Such incidents are not uncommon if your partner has Asperger syndrome, so it is always a good idea to look deeper into any situation. You may not always find a reason, but it is worth checking things out because you may just get to the bottom of it.

What about verbal abuse?

Physical violence was quite uncommon among the women I contacted, but what if the abuse is verbal?

Words can be used in an abusive way and hurt as much as physical abuse.

They can wreck a person's self-esteem and feelings of worth. Episodes of verbal abuse were reported in some of the relationships and, among these, some said this happened quite frequently. Unfortunately, once a pattern of verbal abuse has been established within a couple, it can be very hard to break. This can be even more the case when the abusive partner has Asperger syndrome.

Some change can be achieved if the partner with Asperger syndrome has enough incentive to do something about it, and if you are on the receiving end of such abuse, you need to decide what you are prepared to accept and not accept.

Being objective

Choose an appropriate moment and try to discuss with your partner how what he is saying makes you feel. Alternatively, try writing to your partner if you feel this would have a better effect. A list of words which are not acceptable should be made as well as a list of alternative harmless words. Ask your partner to also draw up such lists.

You should, if possible, try to discuss things in an objective way, remaining neutral and practical. You could try negotiating by saying, 'When you say this to me it makes me upset. If I am upset I cannot cook your dinner, or I cannot talk to you about (special interest). I would be much happier if you would not say ... .'

It is important not to blame or criticise. Your partner also needs to know that what he is saying and doing is all right, even great, and how happy it makes you when he does this or says that. You should both try to keep in mind the positives about each other and the relationship you share.

Tight boundaries

It is important that your partner knows how his behaviour makes you feel. You should always try to talk about the things that bother you and should not cover up for any behaviour that is in any way abusive as this will give your partner the message that it is OK.

It is not wise to think that your partner just needs to get things out of his system as he may interpret this as being given permission to continue what he is doing. The boundaries must be kept tight, with no fuzzy edges. Those with Asperger syndrome need rules and boundaries because they do not always automatically know what is required of them, either in a social, an emotional or intimate situation.

Being clear and precise

You should always make sure that your partner knows exactly which types of behaviour are completely unacceptable and, if possible, let him know this right from the start. He needs to be told what is not acceptable and that the relationship will be at severe risk or, if necessary, finished if he crosses these boundaries.

For those with Asperger syndrome, rules and boundaries must be very clear and precise. It should not be taken for granted that your partner will understand automatically from the beginning what is acceptable and what is not. A lot will depend on his own parental role models and what kind of upbringing he had, as habits and messages that Asperger syndrome children pick up at an early age can be very difficult to challenge and change.

The importance of early diagnosis

If you met at a relatively young age and recognised pretty soon that your partner had Asperger syndrome or if a positive diagnosis was given early on and he received the help and guidance required, then there is a far better chance of making your relationship work and being able to compromise and negotiate together. The ways in which your partner will interact socially and communicate will be learnt behaviour rather than an automatic reaction to any given two-way interaction, but it will be presented quite convincingly.

If, however, the diagnosis was not made until late, possibly with a failed marriage already behind him, it will be more difficult to change things because your partner will already be quite set in his ways and have developed set routines. He may have developed certain 'scripts' and patterns for different situations – even a very set script for what is a 'wife' or 'husband'. This might be based on his experience of how his mother and father played out their relationship, something he has read or watched on television or maybe his relationship with a previous partner. Bringing about change in these circumstances can be harder but, with an awareness of what is causing the difficulties and an incentive to try to change things, the relationship can still improve.

STAYING TOGETHER

The positive sides of Asperger syndrome

Many of the women I contacted attribute all the positive qualities their partner displays to his own individual personality. For some women the main plus point they mention is their partner's gentleness – they feel safe in the knowledge that he is unlikely to ever become violent or hurt them. For others, the most positive thing about them is their faithfulness and the way they do not flirt or appear interested in others sexually. This makes them feel secure and, for many women, being able to relax and be themselves rather than feeling threatened by other women is a great bonus. Others said that they are pleased that their partner is not 'one of the boys', does not live at the pub and come in drunk at night. They like the fact that their partner is far happier to stay in at home, watching the television or working on the house.

Things can get better in time

It does seem that people with Asperger syndrome improve with age and, with time, the negative aspects of the syndrome can lessen. This may happen because they learn more about what their partner wants and does not want. They also want a quiet life and this need probably increases as they get older, so they learn that if they do x, y will happen. This does not mean they are getting over Asperger syndrome, just that they are learning strategies to avoid annoying anyone and making their life with their partner easier. It may also be that their partner is becoming more familiar with the syndrome and possibly echoing some Asperger traits themselves. Although it might seem as if this would make the relationship more manageable, it can leave their partner feeling that they have lost part of themselves.

Taking on Asperger traits

If, after a period of time, you start to wonder if you have Asperger syndrome yourself or are developing Asperger traits, then you really have to think seriously what you are going to do about it, as you could end up feeling that you have lost your individuality or 'self'. A sense of self is important for any individual who wishes to remain an individual, so maybe this is a sign that you need to start doing more for yourself or spending more time in the company of those who do not have Asperger syndrome. If you do not have many friends, then you could take up a hobby that involves others, such as art classes or a part-time course. Maybe you could take a short break with a good friend or the children. Whatever you decide on, it must bring you into contact with other people who do not have Asperger syndrome.

Self-help

Many of the women in relationships with someone with Asperger syndrome display a strong ability to make changes in their lives in order to improve things for themselves. Some go to counselling or seek some other form of therapeutic help – yoga, an exercise class and so on. Others take up some form of studying, and enrol at their local college or university as mature students and discover they have talents they did not know existed. Many create a support system and lives for themselves outside the relationship so that they do not depend solely on him for emotional support, which they have realised he is unable to give them.

All of the women I contacted in my research have, in some way, taken control of their situation and done something positive about it. If you are in this situation, then you are doing something positive about your situation by reading this book.

If one of you decides to leave

It would be quite unusual for your partner to be the one to walk out on your relationship. If he did decide to leave, however, it would be a rare thing if he came back, and if he did, it would probably be on his terms with you as the one who would make most of the changes.

If the partner with Asperger syndrome leaves, clearly it can be devastating for the abandoned partner who is left in a state of shock, wondering how her partner could do this to her when she has tried so hard. It could be helpful at this time for the partner to find a counsellor who understands and can help them through this difficult time.

It could be equally devastating for the partner with Asperger syndrome to be abandoned, and many women expressed the concern that they felt their partners would not be able to cope without them. Everyone has choices. We can decide to stay in a relationship or leave. Every man and woman in our society has that choice. It is not enough to stay for the children or financial reasons or because one partner has become dependent on the other, if the cost is a loss of well-being, self-esteem and health.

A partner with Asperger syndrome can give a lot, but there are some things he will not be able to give. There are some ways in which he can change, but there are also some things he will not be able to change. Your partner is quite capable of loving someone, but may not be very good at showing or expressing it. Neither will he always be able to offer you suitable emotional support or make you feel you are understood and are receiving adequate empathy.

Some women reported feeling that their partner's love for them felt more like a need, that they felt important to them for many reasons but not because they needed a soul mate who could share their deepest feelings and most intimate secrets. It is quite possible to feel that you are needed in the same way that a walking stick is needed by someone who has a limp – that you make your partner's journey through life easier, safer and more comfortable.

Your partner will want you to share his time and special interests. His need for you will be of a very practical and necessary nature but, in return, he will be able to offer you the kind of loyalty that is hard to match.

A special kind of security

Your partner can offer you a special kind of security that, in these days of high rates of divorce and separation, is very hard to find. He will probably stick by you for all of your life. He is very likely to work hard and take care of what he is able to.

Most of the partners with Asperger syndrome whom I interviewed showed a strong commitment to their relationships and offered a sincere faithfulness. Those with Asperger syndrome who are committed and hardworking individuals are generally loyal and long-term partners.

It is up to you to decide what is most important to you. Maybe it is best if you think of your partner as having a disability. This disability restricts him in some areas of social interaction, communication and imaginative thought, but it does not alter the kind of person he is – his morals, level of commitment to the relationship, whether or not he is violent or abusive to you or your children or if he is faithful or not. Your decision to stay or not stay should be based on the things that your partner can make his own decisions about, not just the fact that he has Asperger syndrome.

USEFUL SOURCES OF HELP AND INFORMATION

The Asperger Syndrome Coalition of the United States (ASC-US)
PO Box 351268
Jacksonville, FL 32235-1265
Tel: 864-4-ASPRGR   www.asperger.org

ASC-US is a national, volunteer nonprofit organization comitted to providing information and support services for individuals, families and professionals affected by Asperger syndrome and related disorders such as pervasive developmental disorder/not otherwise specified (PDD-NOS), and high-functioning autism (HFA). ASC-US offers an annual conference and quarterly newsletter.

The Autism Society of America (ASA)
7910 Woodmont Avenue, Suite 300
Bethesda, MD 20814-3067
Tel: 301-657-0881   www.autism-society.org

ASA promotes lifelong access and opportunities for persons within the autism spectrum and their families, to be fully included, participating members of their communities through advocacy, public awareness, education, and research. Their magazine, The Advocate, is distributed internationally.

Maap Services, Inc.
PO Box 524
Crown Point, IN 46308
Tel: 219 662 1311   www.maapservices.org

Maap Services, Inc. was the national organization to focus its efforts on individuals with high-functioning Autism and Asperger syndrome. Founded by Susan Moreno, Maap offers many services including an annual conference with a strand by and for individuals on the spectrum, a quarterly newsletter, and technical support. The Maap newsletter is distributed in 38 countries.

The Asperger Backup Campaign
1 Melville Road
Bournemouth BH9 2PL

The Asperger Backup Campaign (A.B.C.) is a support network for families affected by Asperger syndrome in the Bournemouth area. Brenda Wall runs the A.B.C. alone and can offer limited help and advice to partners, parents and children of people with Asperger syndrome living locally.

Derby Relate Line
Tel: 01332 345678 lines open every Tuesday, 10.30am until 4.30pm

The NAS has developed and delivered a suitable training package for trained counsellors at Derby Relate and the telephone service was launched in 2000. The Derby Relate line enables you to talk directly to a counsellor and discuss, in confidence, any relationship issues you have regarding Asperger syndrome. All calls to the Derby Relate Line are charged at the standard national rate.

Families of Adults Afflicted with Asperger Syndrome
PO Box 514 Centerville
MA 02632   www.faaas.org

The FAAAS support group is run by Karen E. Rodman, whose husband has both Asperger and Tourette's syndromes. Because of the world-wide interest in adults with Asperger syndrome, FAAAS is in the planning stages of opening chapters and districts across the USA and internationally as well.

The National Autistic Society
Head Office
393 City Road
London EC1V 1NG
Tel: 020 7833 2299   www.nas.org.uk

The NAS is the UK's foremost charity for people with autism and Asperger syndrome, and for their parents and caregivers. The NAS leads national and international initiatives providing a strong voice for autism. The organisation works in many areas to help people with an autism spectrum disorder live their lives with as much independence as possible.

FURTHER READING

Attwood, Tony (1998) *Asperger Syndrome: a guide for parents and professionals.*
London: Jessica Kingsley.

Baron-Cohen, Simon (1997) *Mindblindness: an essay on autism and theory of mind.*
London: MIT Press.

Frith, Uta (ed.) (1991) *Autism and Asperger syndrome.*
Cambridge: Cambridge University Press.

Ratey, John J., and Johnson, Catherine (1998) *Shadow syndromes.*
New York: Bantam Books

Schopler, Eric, Mesibov, Gary B., and Kunce, Linda L. (1998) *Asperger syndrome or high-functioning autism.* New York: Plenum Press.

Tantam, Digby, and Prestwood, Sue, S. (1999) *A mind of one's own.*
London: The National Autistic Society (3rd edn).

Willey, Liane Holliday (1999) *Pretending to be normal.*
London: Jessica Kingsley.

Wing, Lorna (1996) *The Autistic spectrum: a guide for parents and professionals.*
London: Constable.

REFERENCES

1. American Psychiatric Association (1994) *Diagnostic and statistical manual of mental disorders* (4th ed.), Washington DC.

2. Asperger, H. (1944) Die 'Autistischen Psychopath' im Kindesalter, *Archiv für psychiatrie und nervenkrankheiten*, 117, pp.76–136, reprinted in U. Frith (1991) *Autism and Asperger syndrome*, Cambridge University Press.

3. Attwood, T. (1998) *Asperger's syndrome: a guide for parents and professionals*, Jessica Kingsley.

4. Bailey, A., et al. (1995), 'Autism as a strongly genetic disorder: evidence from a British twin study', *Psychological Medicine*, 25, pp.63–77.

5. Baron-Cohen, S., and Wheelwright, C. S. (1999) ' "Obsessions" in children with Autism or Asperger syndrome', *British Journal of Psychiatry*, 175, pp.484–90.

6. Baron-Cohen, S., et al. (1997) 'Is there a link between engineering and autism?', *Autism*, 1, pp.101–9.

7. Burgoine, E., and Wing, L. (1983) 'Identical triplets with Asperger's syndrome', *British Journal of Psychiatry*, 143, pp.261–5.

8. Ehlers, S., and Gillberg, C. (1993) 'The epidemiology of Asperger syndrome — A total population study', *Journal of Child Psychology and Psychiatry*, 34, pp.1327–50.

9. Folstein, S. E., et al (1998) 'Finding specific genes that cause Autism: a combination of approaches will be needed to maximize power', *Journal of Autism and Developmental Disorders*, 28(5), pp.439–45.

10. Gillberg, C. (1989) 'Asperger syndrome in 23 Swedish children', *Developmental Medicine and Child Neurology*, 31, pp.520–31.

11. Gillberg, C. (1991) 'Clinical and neurobiological aspects of Asperger syndrome in six family studies', in Uta Frith. (ed.) (1991) *Autism and Asperger syndrome*, Cambridge University Press.

12. Kadesjö, B., Gillberg, C., and Hagberg, B. (1999) 'Brief report: Autism and Asperger syndrome in seven-year-old children: a total population study', *Journal of Autism and Developmental Disorders*, 29 (4), pp.327–31.

13. Noller, P. (1980) 'Misunderstandings in marital communication: a study of couples' non-verbal communication', *Journal of Personality and Social Psychology*, 39, pp.1135–48.

14. Schopler, E., Mesibov, G. B., and Kunce, L. J. (1998) *Asperger syndrome or high-functioning Autism?*, Plenum Press.

15. Then, D., (1997) *Women who stay with men who stray*, Thorsons.

16. Willey, L. H. (1999) *Pretending to be normal*, Jessica Kingsley.

17. Wing. L. (1981) 'Asperger's Syndrome: a clinical account', *Psychological Medicine*, 11, pp.115–30.

INDEX